HEINEMANN MEDICAL
STUDEN

CLINICAL

7.95

Series editor: Professor Peter Richards MA, MD, PhD, FRCP
Professor of Medicine and Dean, St Mary's Hospital Medical School, London

Other titles in the series:
Cancer
Community Medicine: A Study Guide
Geriatric Medicine
Medicine and the Law
Primary Care
Psychology and Medicine

Heinemann Medical
Student Reviews

Clinical Nutrition

GRAHAM NEALE
MA, BSc, MB, ChB, FRCP
Consultant Physician, Addenbrooke's Hospital, and
Honorary Consultant in Clinical Nutrition,
MRC Dunn Nutrition Unit, Cambridge

Heinemann Medical Books
London

Heinemann Medical Books
22 Bedford Square
London WC1B 3HH

ISBN 0-433-23070-3

© Graham Neale, 1988

First published 1988

British Library Cataloguing-in-Publication Data

Neale, Graham
 Clinical nutrition.—(Heinemann
 medical student reviews).
 1. Nutrition
 I. Title
 612'.3   RA784

 ISBN 0-433-23070-3

Typeset by Wilmaset, Birkenhead, Wirral
and printed in Great Britain by Biddles Ltd, Guildford

Contents

	Preface	vii
1	Dietary intake	1
2	Nutrition in growth and development	20
3	Nutritional assessment	42
4	Recognition and management of nutritional disorders	83
5	Nutritional support	132
6	Diet and the epidemiology of disease	168
7	The future of clinical nutrition	191
	Appendix 1: General further reading	204
	Appendix 2: Training and career opportunities	206
	Index	208

Preface

Clinical nutrition does not exist as a specialty in the National Health Service; everyone is involved. Physicians care for patients with nutritionally-determined disorders: endocrinologists for diabetics, for those with metabolic bone disease and for the obese; gastroenterologists for patients with malnutrition secondary to intestinal disease; paediatricians for premature babies, for infants with feeding problems and for those with inborn errors of metabolism; and geriatricians for the ill-nourished elderly. Surgeons are responsible for most patients requiring total parenteral nutrition; obstetricians are concerned with the nutritional requirements during pregnancy and general practitioners are faced with the endless stream of questions from their patients regarding the interaction of diet and disease.

So why try to cover clinical nutrition in a single book? Professor Peter Richards, Dean of St Mary's Hospital Medical School, persuaded me that it was a 'black hole' in the curriculum and that newly qualified doctors were all too ready to push away nutritional problems as the concern of dietitians. In my experience he is right. Yet surely in clinical medicine the ultimate test of a theme worthy of study is its application to and importance for the management of patients. The subject matter of *Clinical Nutrition* appears to fulfil these criteria. Patients in hospital often show the adverse nutritional effects of prolonged cardiac insufficiency, of the major neoplastic diseases and of severe gastrointestinal pathology. Frequently, clinicians see the need to provide nutritional support for patients undergoing major surgery, or encounter the nutritionally-related metabolic disorders induced by alcohol, renal failure, liver failure and pancreatic disease. In addition, doctors are increasingly conscious of those frailties of the elderly which may be nutritionally determined.

In an effort to fill a gap in medical education, this is a book about practical aspects of clinical nutrition by a clinician for clinicians.

Whatever his special interest the clinician should be able to take an adequate dietary history, to determine disorders likely to cause malnutrition, to recognize the signs of disease which may be nutritionally determined, and to work with support services in ordering and interpreting the results of special investigations. He should be familiar with the design of ordinary and therapeutic diets (the dietitian will provide the details) and he needs a detailed knowledge of the most appropriate means of providing artificial nutritional support. He must know how to use pharmaceutical preparations effectively and be aware of the interaction of drugs with nutritional status. Finally he should be able to advise the patient and the patient's family on the principles of sound nutritional practice and to give an informed opinion about the latest dietary fad or pronouncements from specialist committees.

The text starts with a discussion of dietary intake and nutritional assessment before considering the management of nutritional disorders in clinical practice. It is assumed that the reader has a reasonable working knowledge of the principles of physiology and biochemistry which are used to solve clinical problems. Considerable space is given to the practice of artificial nutritional support because the day-to-day management of this important mode of therapy is usually left to junior clinical staff. A chapter is devoted to the potential for preventing premature degenerative disease by nutritional means. This is a subject which no practising clinician can easily avoid because the general public are increasingly well-informed or mis-informed about nutritional matters. The book concludes with a chapter on future possibilities and career opportunities for the clinician interested in nutrition.

Other health professionals may find this clinical approach to nutritional problems of interest. This may be true for dietitians who are concerned with the nutritional management of disease processes (see Chapter 4) and the role of nutrition in preventive medicine (see Chapter 6), for specialist nurses involved in providing artificial nutrition support (see Chapter 5), and for human nutritionists needing background information on nutritionally-related clinical disorders.

I would like to express my thanks to those who have taught me and have encouraged my interest in clinical nutrition. I owe a special debt of gratitude to Sir Christopher Booth at the Royal Postgraduate Medical School; Peter Gatenby, Donald Weir and John Scott in Dublin; Philip James, John Cummings and Marinos Elia at the MRC Dunn Clinical Nutrition Centre, Cambridge; the Nutrition Team at Addenbrooke's Hospital and the many physicians and surgeons with whom I have

Preface

worked. This book would not have been written without the stimulus, support and gentle nagging of Professor Peter Richards and the encouragement of Dr Richard Barling of Heinemann Medical Books. Finally, I thank my wife, Rosemary, for constructive help in putting the subject matter together and for typing the manuscript.

(Throughout the book the clinician has been referred to as 'he' and the dietitian as 'she', and it should be noted that this has been done for reasons of clarity and convenience only.)

Graham Neale

Chapter 1

Dietary Intake

WORLD FOOD • A HISTORICAL PERSPECTIVE • ASSESSMENT OF DIETARY INTAKE • DIETARY HISTORY IN CLINICAL PRACTICE • THE FUTURE • FURTHER READING

In the first half of this century clinical nutrition was largely about the deficiency disorders; xerophthalmia, beri-beri, pellagra, rickets, scurvy, iron deficiency and goitre were all recognized as clinical disorders occurring largely as a result of inadequate dietary intake. Slowly, however, it was recognized that good nutrition is not simply a matter of providing enough. The disappearance of pellagra from the USA was not due simply to the enrichment of cereals with vitamin B; the appearance of rickets in Asian children in the UK has not been due solely to vitamin D deficiency.

An artificial chemical diet has been devised on which adult humans can live in apparently good health for at least several weeks (Table 1.1). We know the required components but translating them into an optimal dietary intake remains a central problem for nutritional scientists. A century ago Voit stated that 'a normal diet is a well-tasting mixture of foodstuffs in proper quantity and in such proportions as to least burden the organism'. In practice this has been translated into the need to build up a diet from a mixture of four food categories:

- meats and pulses
- fruit and vegetables
- dairy products
- cereals and bread

Some authorities include a fifth group of 'calories-only' food, which may be used to satisfy any residual energy gap. In practice dietary intake varies enormously from region to region, from country to country and from rich to poor living in the same environment.

Table 1.1 A chemically defined diet for a sedentary adult man (amounts per day) (after Olson, 1978)

Substance	Amount	Substance	Amount	Substance	Amount
Water	1800 ml	Calories		Bulk	
		Glucose	600 g	Cellulose	20 g
Minerals		Amino acids		Vitamins	
Ammonium acetate	20.8 g	L-Leucine	1.1 g	Ascorbic acid	100 mg
Calcium acid phosphate	5.0 g	L-Methionine	1.1 g	Vitamin E	20 mg
Sodium chloride	3.0 g	L-Phenylalanine	1.1 g	Niacin	20 mg
Potassium chloride	3.0 g	L-Lysine	0.8 g	Pantothenate	10 mg
Magnesium carbonate	1.0 g	L-Valine	0.8 g	Pyridoxine	3.5 mg
Zinc sulphate	50 mg	L-Isoleucine	0.7 g	Riboflavin	2.5 mg
Ferrous sulphate	20 mg	L-Tryptophan	0.3 g	Thiamin	1.5 mg
Manganese sulphate	10 mg	L-Threonine	0.5 g	Vitamin A	1.0 mg
Sodium silicate	10 mg			Vitamin K	0.1 mg
Chromium sulphate	5 mg	Fatty acids		Folate	0.1 mg
Nickel sulphate	5 mg	Trilinolein	5.0 g	Biotin	0.1 mg
Sodium selenate	5 mg			Vitamin D	0.01 mg
Copper sulphate	5 mg			Vitamin B12	0.01 mg
Sodium fluoride	2 mg				
Sodium molybdate	2 mg				
Stannic sulphate	1 mg				
Potassium iodide	1 mg				
Sodium vanadate	0.1 mg				

Olson R. E. (1978). Clinical nutrition, an interface between human ecology and internal medicine. *Nut. Rev;* **36**: 161–77.

WORLD FOOD

Man is able to adapt to a wide range of dietary intake. Cereals dominate the world food supply providing 85% of the total staples. If supplies are adequate, wheat, rice and millet contain just about enough protein to meet minimal needs but maize is deficient in the essential amino acids tryptophan and lysine. In parts of Africa where cassava or plantain are the chief source of energy (see Table 1.7) protein intake may be seriously deficient.

Thus the staple diet must be supplemented by at least some food of a higher protein content. Meat and dairy produce are plentiful in temperate regions, but supplies are limited in most tropical and subtropical countries. People in these areas are often dependent on pulses and groundnuts to supplement their protein intake, especially if fish is unavailable. In contrast, in the cold temperate and arctic regions, fish and sea mammals are important sources of food. The range of human diet is considerable (Table 1.2) and it is not surprising that dietary intake has been correlated with geographic patterns of disease (see Chapter 6).

Protein intake per capita ranges from less than 40 to more than 90 g/day and energy from less than 2000 to more than 3000 kcal (8400–12 500 kJ)/day (Fig. 1.1). Within countries there are extraordinary variations in the availability of food (Table 1.3). The poor, particularly women and children, bear the brunt of underconsumption. Of people in the developing world, 25% are seriously undernourished (United Nations World Conference on the Food Situation, 1985) with the greatest concentration of malnutrition in central Africa.

The energy needs of man are not clearly defined. The US National Academy of Sciences has progressively reduced its estimates of the needs for a moderately active 70 kg man from 3000 kcal (12.5 MJ) in 1943 and 3200 kcal (13.4 MJ) in 1950 to 2800 kcal (11.6 MJ) in 1968 and 2700 kcal (10.3 MJ) in 1974. The FAO/WHO figures of recommended intake in 1973 were 3000 kcal (12.5 MJ) for a working man weighing 65 kg and 2200 kcal (9.20 MJ) for a woman of 55 kg. These figures were based on an observed averaged intake by apparently healthy subjects in developed western countries. In Papua New Guinea, Norgan (1974) showed that healthy adult males (56 kg) living an easy life on the coast consume less than 2000 kcal (8.4 MJ) in contrast to the 2500 kcal (10.5 MJ) ingested by apparently equally healthy hardworking people of similar weight in the highlands. Overall energy

Table 1.2 Global variations in sources of energy and protein

Region	Dietary energy intake	Protein intake Vegetable	Protein intake Animal	Intake kcal	Intake Protein
Western world	CHO (80 g sucrose/lactose) Fat 100 g		Mainly meat/dairy produce	2750+	100 g+
Mediterranean	CHO (esp. pasta) Fat 75 g (esp. vegetable oil) Alcohol		Mixed	2200+	70 g
India	CHO (rice/wheat) 200–300 g	Pulses/beans 25 g	Dairy produce 10 g	1500	50 g
China	CHO (rice/wheat) 500 g	Mixed vegetables 20 g	Animal protein 7 g	2500	70 g
Central America	CHO (maize) 500 g	Beans 20 g	Variable	2400	70 g
East Africa (Mozambique)	CHO (cassava/maize) 250 g	Pulses 20 g	Variable	1300	30–40 g

Table 1.3 World food availability per person by region 1961 and 1984

Country	Energy (kcal/MJ)			Protein (g)			Fat (g)		
	1961	1984	(change)	1961	1984	(change)	1961	1984	(change)
North America, north west Europe	3100/13	3450/14.5	(+10%)	90	105	(+15%)	100	130	(+30%)
Central and south America	2350/10	2600/11	(+10%)	60	65	(+5%)	50	60	(+20%)
North Africa	2100/9	2800/12	(+35%)	60	75	(+25%)	40	65	(+60%)
South-east Asia	1850/7.5	2100/9	(+15%)	40	55	(+30%)	25	35	(+40%)
China/east Asia	1800/7.5	2800/12	(+55%)	45	65	(+50%)	15	40	(+150%)
West and central Africa	2100	2100	(...)	50	55	(+10%)	40	40	(...)

Source: FAO estimates July 1986.
Data abstracted from: *The State of the World's Children*. (1987). Published for UNICEF by Oxford University Press, Oxford.

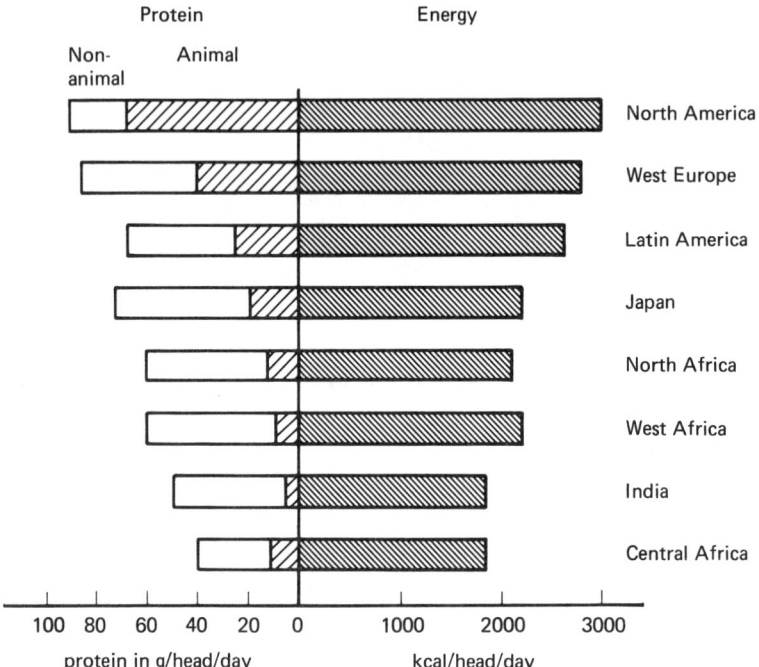

Figure 1.1 Food availability per head of population (at a global level). (Data drawn from Lapedes D. N., editor in chief. (1977). *Encyclopedia of Food, Agriculture and Nutrition.* New York, London: McGraw Hill.) 1 kcal ≈ 4.2 kJ.

requirements depend on several variables (Table 1.4). In assessing published data, it is important to remember that recommended dietary allowances (RDAs) are those considered adequate for at least 95% of the population, i.e. 2 SD above the mean. Many people live, apparently healthily, on much less. In contrast, in affluent societies, man adapts to a diet which contains more calories than he requires, much food of animal origin and considerable amounts of refined carbohydrate.

The problem of undernutrition

Malnutrition has multiple causes (Table 1.5). It cannot be ascribed simply to underproduction, overpopulation and poor distribution.

Dietary Intake

Table 1.4 *Factors affecting human energy requirements*

Body weight
Body composition
Physical activity
Metabolic characteristics
Diet

Basal metabolic rate in the habitually 'underfed' is 10–30% below that of the well-fed.

Table 1.5 *Socioeconomic factors associated with widespread undernutrition*

Low food production
    Drought and crop failures
Poverty
    Unable to afford seed, fertiliser, equipment and energy (oil)
Poor sanitation
    Communicable disease
Illiteracy
    Slow to learn new methods
Population pressure
Uneven distribution wealth
    Unemployment
    Social diseases

In coping with the problem of widespread undernutrition, attempts are now being made to promote self-sufficiency, whereas previously the emphasis was on producing food for market. Thus resources have been poured into the more fertile areas worked by commercial methods with high energy costs (Table 1.6) and this has aggravated the problems of subsistence for peasant farmers, especially in tropical and subtropical lands. In such areas, 60 to 80% of the adult population is directly involved in agriculture. Taking the better land for food production is often disastrous. Dispossessed farm workers migrate to the towns and subsist in the best way they can. The problem is aggravated by the silent demographic revolution; in Third World countries, the death rate has fallen dramatically with little change in the birth rate. The energy costs

Table 1.6 The energy efficiency of food production

Food	Energy ratio: (energy produced/ energy expended)	Relative output (per unit area)
Rice (China)	40	Very high
Maize (Africa)	40	Moderate
Cereals and roots (shifting cultivation)	20	Very low
Groundnuts (Africa)	12	Moderate
Maize (USA)	2.5	High
Wheat (UK)	2.5	High
Sugar (Europe)	0.7	High
Cattle (farm)	0.7	Low
Sheep (farm)	0.25	Very low
Poultry/eggs (farm)	0.15	Low

Data abstracted from Leah G. (1976). *Energy and Food Production.* London: IPC Science and Technical Press.

associated with food production, summarized in Table 1.6, clearly illustrates the differences in industrialized systems. The pre-industrialized systems use human labour and animal power, and the main energy input is food; semi-industrialized systems, where some of the crop is marketed, use machinery and fertilizers. The fully industrialized systems are highly dependent on machinery, fertilizers and pesticides. In combined crop–animal systems most of the crop is fed to animals in order to produce high protein food for humans. In fully industrialized cropping, therefore, high energy input is needed.

In Third World countries, the present WHO strategy is to produce programmes which will broaden the food base using indigenous crops (Table 1.7), adapt to the differing roles of men and women in the production and preparation of food, and take account of rapidly evolving socioeconomic conditions. The overall aim is to develop technologies which are ecologically sound, economically viable and culturally acceptable. The task is enormous. And there is a major role for nutritionally trained scientists to monitor the results of their efforts.

Nutrition in affluent countries

In most parts of the Western World people can afford to eat largely that which pleases their palates. Nutritionists struggle to produce guidelines

Dietary Intake

Table 1.7 Some of the more important food crops of tropical Africa

Indigenous crops	Imported from Asia	Imported from America
Cereal		
Sorghum	Wheat	Maize
Millet	Barley	
West African rice	Rice	
Legumes and pulses		
Cowpea	Pea	Common bean
Horse-eye bean	Lentil	
	Soya bean	
Roots and tubers		
Yam	Taro	Potato
Kaffir potato	Greater yam	Sweet potato
Yam bean		Cassava
Fruits		
Tamarind	Banana	Pineapple
Desert date	Plantain	Avocado
African mango	Citrus	Guava
Water melon	Mango	Passion fruit
Green vegetables		
African spinach	Eggplant	Chilli
Bitterleaf	Pepper	Tomato
Fluted pumpkin	Ginger	Pumpkin
Elephant grass	Onion	
Oil plants		
Bambara groundnut	Coconut	Groundnut
Oil palm	Safflower	Cashew
Sesame		
Breadfruit		
Castor bean		
Sugar	Sugar cane	

for what is often termed a 'balanced diet' – a diet which contains the 'correct' amounts and 'correct' ratios of nutrients (see Bender and Bender, 1982).

In 1977 the US Senate published *Dietary goals for the United States*. Essentially this was a programme for the prevention of atheroma and its complications (heart attacks, peripheral vascular disease and strokes) and for decreasing the incidence of cancer, diabetes and cirrhosis of the liver. More recently in the UK, the report of the National Advisory Committee on Nutrition Education (NACNE) made similar if more cautious proposals (Table 1.8). Both publications produced violent reactions. On the one hand there were activists who sought action by the government to prevent the 'new epidemic' of disease caused by modern diets, on the other hand the more cautious scientists were opposed to the publication of recommendations without better scientific evidence and properly conducted clinical trials. However, the major protest against the dietary recommendations came from agricultural interests and the food industry. Clearly manufacturers have a vested interest in producing food cheaply and profitably, some without too much regard for the possible long-term implications for health. Moreover food is big business. The organizations involved are not short of money for advertising, have uncountable market outlets and a diffuse network of retailers. It is not surprising that on occasions the industry as a whole is accused of unscrupulous behaviour. Nevertheless professional nutritionists should be careful of not biting the hand that feeds. They must be aware that it is not easy for farmers and food manufacturers to respond quickly to changes in fashion. Overproduction is a recurring nightmare for farmers and contamination of preserved foods either chemically or bacteriologically may have disastrous consequences for the organizations which prepare and package much of what we eat. The national diet reflects the balance between human taste (I eat it because I like it) the advice of nutritionists (I eat it because it is good for me) and the market place economy (I eat it because it is cheap and convenient). The public are bombarded with information but this is only one factor affecting the evolution of national eating habits (see Fig. 1.2, p. 12).

How these changes will influence the prevalence of disease is difficult to determine because the major diseases of the Western World have a complex aetiology. Indeed a prominent American nutritional scientist, Olson, stated in 1978 that 'a trade-off in disease morbidity for every major change in diet is not inevitable but is probable'.

A HISTORICAL PERSPECTIVE

Attempts have been made to estimate the dietary intake of primitive man on the grounds that this represents the nutrition to which humans are best adapted – the so-called 'Stone Age diet'. It is agreed that coronary artery disease, hypertension, diabetes and some forms of cancer are diet-related, and that these disorders are rarely seen in the

Dietary Intake

Table 1.8 *Proposals for long-term changes in the British diet by the National Advisory Committee on Nutrition Education*

1.	Dietary recommendations should be applicable to the whole population
2.	Goals to be based on the most beneficial average intake (rather than on defined limits)
3.	Energy intake to be defined in terms of optimal body weight and adequate exercise
4.	To be reaffirmed that the risks of smoking far exceed the risks of obesity
5.	*Fat* Decrease from about 38% to about 30% total energy intake*
6.	*Saturated fatty acid* Decrease from about 18% to 10% total energy intake*
7.	*Sucrose* Decrease from 40 to 20 kg/year
8.	*Fibre* Increase from 20 to 30 g/day
9.	*Salt* Decrease by 3 g/day (actual intake uncertain 8–12 g/day)
10.	*Alcohol* Decrease from approximately 7% to 4% energy intake
11.	*Protein* No change (but greater proportion from vegetables)
12.	*Minerals and vitamins* As recommended dietary allowance (RDA)
13.	Recommendations apply to all with only small adjustments for special groups (e.g. need for supplements of vitamin D for Asians eating traditional Indian food)
14.	Foods to be more fully labelled

*No recommendations for:
5. Cholesterol intake.
6. Polyunsaturated: saturated fatty acids (P:S Ratio).
It is recognised that there is no clear recommendation from current scientific opinion, and that implementation of the other dietary recommendations will lead to a fall in the intake of cholesterol and a rise in the P:S ratio.

few primitive hunter–gatherer populations surviving today. However, the basis of the argument for the Stone Age diet is not necessarily sound. Observations in primitive people are few, and only a small percentage of such people reach the age of 60 years. Moreover, the diet of early man was far from uniform. The early hominids lived primarily on fruits, nuts, beans and roots. The eating of meat first occurred about 2 million years ago and became a dominant part of the diet 30 000–40 000 years ago. The meat-eaters grew big and strong. Subsequently the climate changed and there was a period of overpopulation. Big game were in short supply and mankind moved to a less attractive form of subsistence living based on a diet of small animals and a variety of plant foods.

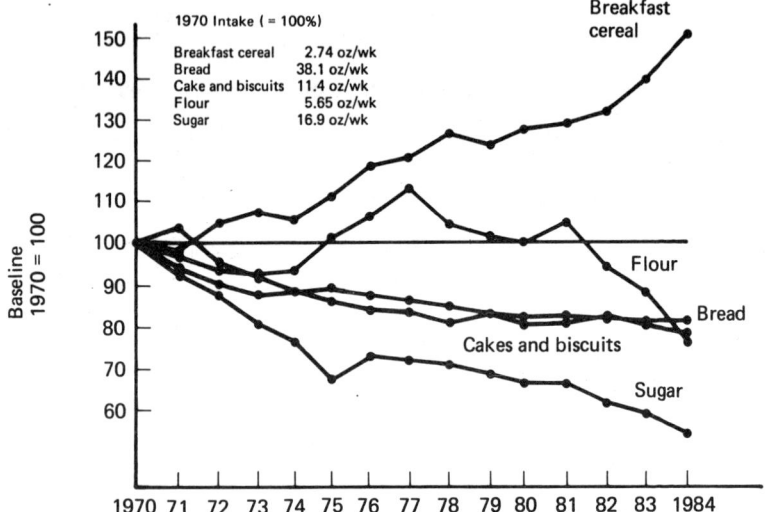

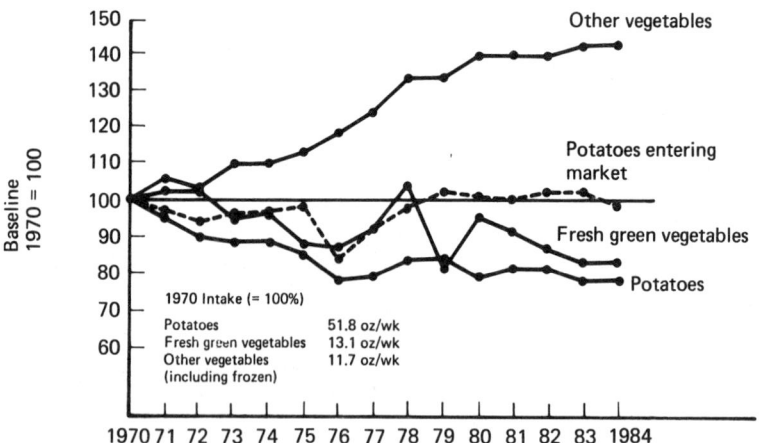

Figure 1.2 Household consumption of various foods. (Graphs drawn from data taken from *Annual Abstract of Statistics*. (1986). Central Statistical Office. London: HMSO.) 1 oz ≈ 28 g.

Dietary Intake

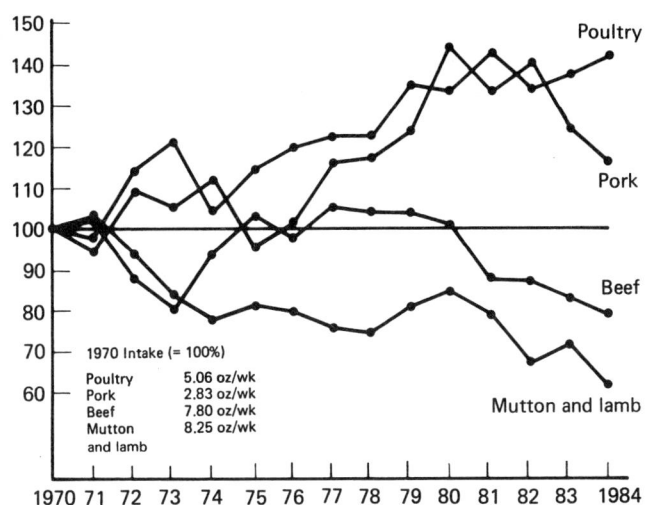

Household consumption of meat 1970-1984

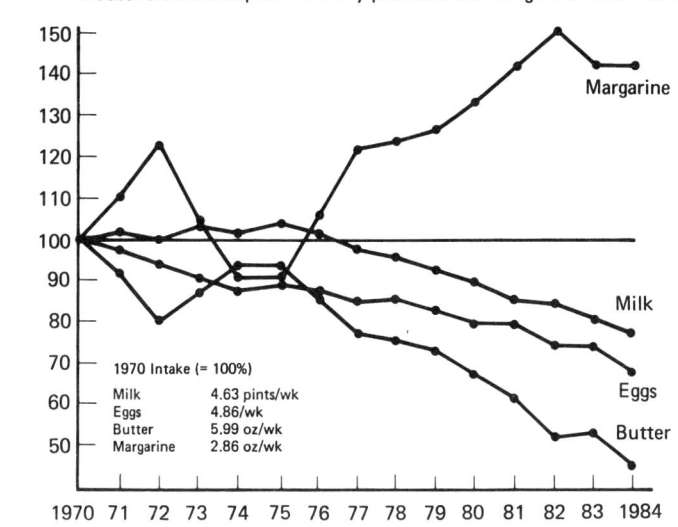

Household consumption of dairy products and margarine 1970-1984

Agriculture developed about 10 000 years ago. In farming areas, vegetable foodstuffs came to comprise 90% or more of the diet, dairying was developed in some areas but not in others. Mankind became considerably shorter with a much less well-developed skeleton. However, the pattern was far from uniform. In some savanna areas big game hunting persisted. In coastal areas, fish formed a significant part of the normal diet and within the Arctic circle the sea provided nearly all the food. The widespread use of cereal grains appeared late in the development of man and only in large quantities after the Agricultural Revolution in the 18th century. Thus the statement that human diseases of the developed world occur because the human genes are poorly programmed for present day diets must be treated with some caution.

Nevertheless, a comparison of the diets of early man with present-day eating habits is thought-provoking. The hunter–gatherer diet probably contained as much cholesterol although much less saturated fat than the average Western diet of today. It may have contained plenty of calcium even without the taking of milk, but almost certainly much less sodium. Vitamins and trace elements were abundant. Despite these differences it is important to remember that diet is only one factor to consider in the development of degenerative disorders. Life-style and exercise may be as important as diet in allowing our genetic make-up to express itself in an optimal way.

ASSESSMENT OF DIETARY INTAKE

Clinicians rarely show much interest in what their patients eat, and even less in what they have been eating. Perhaps this is largely because it is very difficult to demonstrate the relationship between the outcome of a disease process in any one individual and his dietary intake. The clinician is aware of the geographical associations between populations and disease (e.g. for coronary artery disease and colonic cancer) but cannot translate these into cause and effect for an individual patient. To compound the problem the techniques for measuring dietary intake in free-living subjects are unsatisfactory and it is difficult to see how they can be much improved. Yet there are important considerations. The common observation that individuals of the same age, sex and general size may differ substantially in their intake of food and nutrients has been well documented. In 1945 Widdowson and McCance wrote 'One child was always found to be eating twice as much as another of the same age and sex and exactly the same is seen in adults. All the separate dietary constituents varied just as much or more, and one boy of 2 years ate more than a boy of 17.'

Dietary assessment is important in clinical practice, e.g. in managing obesity, diabetes and serious gastrointestinal disorders; in clinical research, e.g. in elucidating the role of sodium in hypertension or in studying the physiology of the colon, and in the wider issues of human economy and epidemiology.

Five methods are commonly used (Table 1.9). The weighed food

Table 1.9 *Methods used for assessing the dietary intake of individuals*

Dietary history and frequency of intake
Dietary recall (previous day—repeated 3 or 4 times)
Dietary diary *(foods and portion sizes recorded)
Weighed intake *(foods and weights recorded)
Duplicate meal preparation and analysis*

*Usually over 7 consecutive days (to include 1 weekend).

record is usually regarded as the gold standard but it is cumbersome and not completely immune from the obvious errors of all methods (Table 1.10). Clinicians rarely attempt to assess the average dietary intake of an individual over a prolonged period. The task is too daunting. Dietary histories taken from control subjects at an interval of 6 months show a correlation of 0.79 for protein and 0.67 for fat. If the interval is 15–25 years the correlation between the diet history taken at the time and that obtained by prolonged recall is usually about 0.25. In contrast, the correlation between the two dietary histories taken at the same time, i.e. present diet : past diet, is of the order of 0.50. The conclusion of the workers providing these data is expressed quite simply: 'the recall of past diets is strongly influenced by present dietary habits'.

DIETARY HISTORY IN CLINICAL PRACTICE

Role of the clinician

A crude assessment of dietary intake is useful in some clinical situations. It is achieved quite simply by asking the patient what he ate the previous day, and how this compares with his usual eating pattern.

Table 1.10 Errors in assessing the food intake of individuals (after Pearson et al., 1982)

Changes in diet induced by
  Observation
  Response to purpose of study
Errors in reporting because of
  Inadequate cooperation
  Defective observation
  Lapses in memory
  Errors in weighing and estimation
Errors in analysis and computation because
  Composition of foods is inconstant
  Table values are only approximate (especially for minerals and vitamins)
  Calculations are tedious (although computer programmes are now available)
Days of weighed intake required to achieve an estimate of average intake to within 10% of 22 days' mean (95% certainty)
  Energy—7 days
  Protein—10 days
  Iron—12 days
  Vitamin C—12 days

Pearson G. C., Morgan D. B., Huppin R. (1982). The period required for a weighed dietary survey of hospitalised patients. *Proc. Nut. Soc.*; **41**: 90A.

Table 1.11 Indirect methods of measuring the dietary intake of free-living subjects when in a steady state

Energy intake	Double-labelled water analysis
Protein intake	Nitrogen excretion
Sodium intake	Sodium excretion
Potassium intake	Potassium excretion

By this method, the clinician may identify a dietary substance which causes symptoms in susceptible subjects. For example, many people are dyspeptic as a result of drinking too much tea or coffee; subjects with hypolactasia may have excess wind and a loose bowel habit after drinking a pint of milk, and occasionally a food substance is found to be the cause of a type I hypersensitivity reaction.

The clinician should also assess the overall dietary pattern. By so doing he may come to suspect inadequate intake of one or more specific

Dietary Intake

nutrients. For example, vitamin B deficiency in the alcoholic who eats poorly, vitamin C deficiency in subjects who avoid vegetables and fruit and vitamin D deficiency in housebound patients who eat no eggs, margarine or fatty fish.

Most people taking specialist diets eat reasonably well-balanced meals. Those who limit variety are most likely to develop deficiencies, such as the vegan who becomes depleted of vitamin B12 because he refuses to take any animal-derived food (see p. 92).

Role of the dietitian

The dietitian is trained to provide a much more accurate assessment of food intake than that obtained by the clinician. Most often she will work from a simple dietary history which she converts into an average intake of calories and specific nutrients. She will be able to spot food fads and possible problems arising from a poorly balanced diet.

In practice, such dietary histories are useful in assessing patients with certain common disorders such as obesity, hyperlipidaemia, weight loss, constipation and suspected food allergy or intolerance.

Occasionally, the dietitian will use the more accurate food diary method. This is particularly helpful in managing some patients with obesity. The discipline of writing down everything eaten for several days is often salutary but the clinician must be wary of the patient who misrepresents dietary habits in order to impress.

For an optimal assessment of food intake the weighing technique must be used. Usually this method is reserved for research projects. The accuracy of the study will depend on the enthusiasm of the observer, the care taken in teaching the subjects and the degree of determination applied to follow-up. In recent epidemiological studies, undertaken by skilled nutritionists, over 70% of randomly-selected adults produced satisfactory data. A check on the accuracy of measured intake is made by determining the urinary excretion of nitrogen and sodium and then comparing output with intake. Checks on urinary excretion of dietary metabolites undertaken some time after a dietary survey appear to confirm that motivated subjects with stable dietary habits do not significantly alter their food intake in response to assessment.

Recently electronic devices have been developed to help the subjects record their food intake. The data obtained is best analysed by computer in order to avoid the tedious arithmetic which has to be applied in order to convert food ingested into nutrient intake.

Table 1.12 Some genetically determined disorders in which careful control of diet may be important in preventing or delaying disease

Disorder	Incidence/prevalence
Uncommon inherited disorders managed primarily by diet	
Amino acid disorders	
Phenylketonuria	1:10 000 births
Maple syrup urine disease	1:100 000 births
Homocystinuria	1:200 000 births
Tyrosinaemia	1:1000 births in localised area French Canada very rare elsewhere
Carbohydrate disorders	
Fructose intolerance	1:20 000 births
Galactosaemia	1:60 000 births
Sucrase-isomaltase deficiency	1:1 000 000 births
Lactase deficiency	Common normal variant
Common genetically-predisposed disorders in which diet important	
Hypercholesterolaemia	25% adults > 250 mg/100 ml
	5% adults > 300 mg/100 ml
	0.2–0.5% population are heterozygotes for monogenic familial disease
Obesity	4% adults Grade 2 (W/H^2 30–40)
(see Chapter 4, Table 4.6, p. 101)	0.05% adults Grade 3 (W/H^2 > 40)
Coeliac disease	1:2000 to 1:10 000 births in Caucasians
Cystic fibrosis	1:2500 births in Caucasians

THE FUTURE

We need to know much more about the dietary habits of individuals. Measurement of body composition, of the excretion of metabolites and of energy output in free-living subjects may provide valuable information (Table 1.11). Ultimately we may be able to assess the effect of diet on the expression of the genome of the ordinary person. The importance of research in this area is seen already in the effective management by diet alone of many rare genetic disorders (Table 1.12).

FURTHER READING

References

Bender A. E., Bender D. A. (1982). *Nutrition for Medical Students.* New York, Chichester: John Wiley.
Central Statistical Office. *Annual Abstract of Statistics.* London: HMSO.
Norgan N. G., Ferro-Luzzi A., Durnin J. (1974). The energy intake in 204 New Ginean adults. *Philos. Trans. Roy. Soc. Lond. (Biol)*; 268: 309–48.
Olson R. E. (1978). Clinical nutrition, an interface between human ecology and internal medicine. *Nut. Rev*; 36: 161–77.
Rosenberg I. H., ed. (1985). Behind and beyond recommended dietary allowances. *Amer. J. Clin. Nut*: 41: 139–70.

General

Blaxter K. (1985). *Technology in the 1990's: Agriculture and Food.* London: Royal Society.
Blaxter K. (1986). *People, Food and Resources.* Cambridge: Cambridge University Press.
Passmore R., Eastwood M. A. (1986). *Human Nutrition and Dietetics*, 8th edn. Edinburgh: Churchill Livingstone.

Assessment of dietary intake

Bingham S. (1987). The dietary assessment of individuals: methods, accuracy, new techniques and recommendations. *Nut. Abst. Rev*; A 57: 705–42.
Lapedes D. N., editor in chief. (1977). *Encyclopaedia of Food, Agriculture and Nutrition.* New York, London: McGraw Hill.
Mahalko J. R., Johnson L. K., Gallagher S. K., Milne D. B. (1985). Comparison of dietary histories and seven-day food records in a nutritional assessment of older adults. *Amer. J. Clin. Nut*; 42: 542–53.
van Staveren W. A., de Boer J. O., Burema J. (1985). Validation and reproducibility of dietary history method estimating the usual food intake during one month. *Amer. J. Clin. Nut*; 42: 554–59.

Chapter 2

Nutrition in Growth and Development

FETAL GROWTH AND DEVELOPMENT • CHILDHOOD • GROWTH AND DEVELOPMENT OF INFANTS • GROWTH AND DEVELOPMENT AT ADOLESCENCE • OPTIMAL GROWTH AND DEVELOPMENT • FURTHER READING

Perinatal and infant mortality are major health concerns in underdeveloped countries and amongst the poor of many industrialized nations. The causes are multifactorial but nutrition is clearly important. Surviving children adapt to their environment. Their growth and development is influenced by the food they eat. But the scientist who seeks to determine diets which will allow the full expression of human intellectual and cultural potential faces many unanswered questions.

FETAL GROWTH AND DEVELOPMENT

Most data on nutritional factors affecting fetal development are related to birth weight. Approximately 7% of babies weigh less than 2500 g at birth. Two-thirds of perinatal deaths are in this group. Morbidity is also closely related to intrauterine growth. Many factors influence birth weight adversely (Table 2.1) and in most studies it is difficult to isolate the effects of undernutrition.

The nutritional cost of pregnancy has been estimated by a factorial method. Moieties are required for the structural and energy requirements of growth, for the increased energy requirements of mother and infant and to provide an energy reserve (body fat increases in most pregnant women) which may be used during lactation.

The total nutritional requirement of pregnancy has been estimated at

Nutrition in Growth and Development

Table 2.1 *Factors which may adversely influence birth weight*

Maternal age
Maternal weight
Socioeconomic status
Infections in pregnancy
? Hard physical work
Tobacco
Alcohol
Malnutrition

Table 2.2 *Metabolic adjustments in the pregnant woman*

Diminished catabolism
Increased proportional absorption of minerals
Increased circulating transport proteins
Active transfer of nutrients across the placenta
Mobilisation of maternal reserves as required
(Protein costs of pregnancy are spread over the whole period of gestation)

80 000 kcals (335 MJ) and 900–1000 g of protein. But this takes little account of the metabolic adjustments which occur in pregnant women (Table 2.2). Observations of the eating habits of pregnant women show that the quantity and quality of the diet can vary widely without obvious impairment of the reproductive process. The increase in food intake is spread throughout pregnancy. There is no dramatic change in the final trimester despite the rapid growth of the fetus at this time. Indeed many women, perhaps most, go through an apparently normal pregnancy with little or no increase in dietary intake. Fetal growth may not be compromised by a diet containing as little as 1600 kcal (6.7 MJ) day. Nutrition intervention studies in underdeveloped countries show that insufficient protein is not normally a limiting factor. In fact there is some evidence to suggest that large protein supplements to poorly nourished pregnant women may lead to an increase in premature deliveries of small infants (as seen in studies of a deprived black population in New York).

Effects of severe undernutrition in pregnancy

In the previous section evidence has been quoted which shows that the fetus is remarkably well protected from maternal food deprivation. Infants born to mothers in rural areas of underdeveloped countries are only marginally smaller than those born to mothers in affluent societies. But starvation has a clearly measurable effect. Women become amenorrhoeic and the birth rate falls. Neonates are on average 10–20% smaller than normal. This was seen in Leningrad during and immediately after the siege of 1941–2, where 50% of term infants weighed less than 2500 g. Conditions in Holland at the end of the Second World War were scarcely any better, and the mean birth weight of full term infants was on average 350 g lower than normal. The weight deficit appeared to be primarily due to reduced body fat. The infants were of normal length and subsequent studies revealed no long-term adverse effects.

Analysis of these clinical observations show that starvation before and during the first trimester adversely affects embryogenesis. Congenital malformations and miscarriages increase. In contrast severe deprivation of food in the last trimester reduces fetal growth and may influence perinatal well-being. If the deprived neonate is subsequently well-fed catch-up growth occurs rapidly and the infant develops normally.

Specific nutrient deficiencies in pregnancy

Deficiencies of specific nutrients in the diets of pregnant women only occasionally cause overt disease in the newborn infant because trace elements and vitamins are actively transferred to the feto–placental unit. Experimentally, however, dietary manipulation may affect fetal development adversely. For example, deficiencies in dietary magnesium or trace elements (e.g. zinc) lead to fetal wastage in rats, as does contamination of the diet with heavy metals (lead, cadmium). These observations are probably not relevant to human pregnancy but some scientists have expressed caution regarding the potential risks of a reduced intake of micronutrients in subjects living largely on processed rather than natural foods.

These data suggest that a good mixed diet without drugs or additives provides the optimal nutritional preparation for a healthy woman seeking to become pregnant. During pregnancy, dietary supplements

Nutrition in Growth and Development

are unnecessary except when there is good reason to expect that the demands of pregnancy will cause significant deficiency in the mother.

Unfortunately it is difficult to predict impending (or even actual) deficiencies of vitamins or trace elements in pregnant women. Normal values or specific nutrients in healthy non-pregnant controls are of little use because of the changes in plasma volume (increased), transport proteins (increased), circulating lipids (increased) and tissue distribution of nutrients. The physiological fall in haemoglobin concentration associated with a downward shift in values for serum iron and folate has led many obstetricians to advise all women to take a pharmaceutical preparation of iron and folic acid throughout pregnancy. Yet there is no convincing evidence that such supplementation confers any advantage to the pregnant woman eating a healthy diet. In affluent countries the desire to help perfect fetal development has led to a detailed examination of nutritional factors but these studies have yielded little in the way of positive results. Pregnancy should be regarded as a physiological occurrence and experimental evidence favours those who preach minimal interference. Certainly fad diets and large supplements of trace elements should not be used.

Iron

The iron requirements of pregnancy are surprisingly poorly defined. The fetus and placenta require rather more than 300 mg but there is uncertainty about the needs for the increased maternal red cell mass. The blood loss on delivery is variable but may be roughly equivalent to the increase in circulating blood cells found at term (equivalent to about 300 mg iron). To meet these needs it is suggested that the pregnant woman needs to absorb an extra 4 mg iron a day during the second half of pregnancy given that she has saved approximately 120 mg by ceasing to menstruate. Normally 1–2 mg iron are absorbed from a mixed diet containing 14 mg per day. Absorption of dietary iron may treble over the 40 weeks of a normal pregnancy. By giving additional inorganic salts, the physiological fall of haemoglobin concentration may be counteracted but this is not necessarily desirable. In practice it is sensible to supplement only those patients at known risk or those who develop overt anaemia.

Zinc

Levels of plasma zinc fall dramatically in pregnancy (to a third of normal). Zinc is a growth factor in experimental animals and zinc deficient diets are believed to be a cause of childhood stunting in some parts of the Middle East. Thus it is not surprising that there is a considerable literature on the zinc requirements of pregnancy. Very low levels of plasma zinc and, perhaps more significantly, white cell zinc have been described in Hindu women bearing low birth weight infants (studies in the UK and the USA). Pharmaceutical supplements of zinc have not been shown to improve birth weight and there is no evidence to show that low zinc levels are associated with congenital malformation or fetal morbidity. Zinc supplements in experimental animals may damage the fetus so should not be given routinely in pregnancy.

Fat-soluble vitamins

Circulating lipids rise in pregnancy, and in healthy women deficiency of fat-soluble vitamins is not a problem. Nevertheless one should heed the possibility of vitamin D deficiency in the management of pregnant women known to have malabsorptive disorders and of those who get poor exposure to sunlight. Neonatal rickets is a rare disorder but it has been described in breast-fed babies and is related to low levels of vitamin D in milk. These can be prevented by giving mothers a small oral supplement of vitamin D (2000 IU/day).

Water-soluble vitamins

The concentration of circulating water-soluble vitamins (including the values for folic acid and vitamin B12) fall in pregnancy without obvious ill-effect. The normal ranges appear to be reset at lower levels. Megaloblastic anaemia is uncommon but should be considered in any pregnant women with significant anaemia, especially if associated with macrocytosis.

The other water-soluble vitamins are not a problem except in countries with endemic malnutrition and theoretically in people who eat very poor diets by choice. There is possibly one important exception to this general rule. Women prone to carry a fetus with a neural tube defect may be sensitive to borderline deficiencies of the water-soluble vitamins (especially folic acid).

Prevention of neural tube defects

Anencephaly, spina bifida and encephalocoele may result from genetic defect, direct intrauterine damage or from an unexplained combination of genetic and environmental factors; 90% of cases are believed to have an environmental component and there are important geographical variations (Europe rather than Asia or Africa; Wales and Ireland rather than south-east England). The genetic component is revealed by the predominance of affected female babies, the 10 fold increase in the incidence of recurrence in siblings, and the ethnic variations.

In 1976, Professor Smithells (Leeds) reported a study of the vitamin status of nearly 1000 women studied during the first trimester of pregnancy (vitamin A, vitamin C, folic acid and riboflavin). The six mothers giving birth to infants with neural tube defects had low levels for all three water-soluble vitamins compared with controls. The results were significant for red cell folate ($p<0.001$) and white cell vitamin C ($p<0.05$). These findings led to two controlled trials of periconceptual vitamin/iron/calcium supplements to mothers who had previously delivered a child with a neural tube defect (NTD). Three tablets of Pregnavite Forte F (Bencard) were given each day for at least 28 days before conception until the second missed menstrual period. Each tablet contained 25 mg iron (as ferrous sulphate), 120 µg folic acid, vitamin B complex (thiamine, riboflavine and pyridoxine), 1333 IU vitamin A, 13.3 mg ascorbic acid, 133 IU vitamin D and 160 mg calcium phosphate. Thus it is impossible to identify a specific active factor. Be that as it may in both trials (the second was multicentre), the recurrence rates for NTD were remarkably lower for mothers taking vitamin supplements (by factors of 3- to 8-fold).

The data look convincing but several observers believe that they are open to more than one interpretation. Much of the criticism is based on the possibility of biassed selection of control and treated groups. Currently the Medical Research Council is trying to resolve the problem by running an independent trial. There are also plans to try to determine whether or not folic acid is as effective as a multivitamin preparation in preventing NTD. Curiously this trial is taking place against a natural fall in the incidence of NTD in England and Wales. The figures have fallen from more than 4 in 1000 births in 1972 to close to 1 in 1000 births in 1984. Prenatal diagnosis and subsequent termination of pregnancy do not account for all the difference and it is difficult to believe that there has been a much improved dietary intake over so short a period. The incidence of NTD has also fallen in the Republic of Ireland where prenatal diagnosis is not available. Thus, although a simple and apparently safe method of reducing NTD may be available, the condition itself remains an enigma.

Alcohol damage

It is now well established that alcohol is teratogenic in humans although in the UK the first cases of deformity were not reported until 1982. Fetal alcohol syndrome (FAS) is characterized by mental deficiency (IQ 50–75), craniofacial malformation and poor growth. Despite its name, the damage occurs primarily during embryogenesis and the fully developed syndrome is only the apex of a range of disorders. In Scandinavia, alcohol ingestion in pregnancy is believed to account for 8% of all cases of mild mental retardation. A recent study in London suggests that an intake of as little as 10 g alcohol a day (a pint of beer, a glass of wine) in early pregnancy may double the individual risk of producing a baby weighing less than 2500 g at birth.

The measurement of behavioural variables in the infants of mothers taking alcohol regularly suggest a dose-response rather than a threshold effect. The most obvious damage to cerebral function concerns the central processing of information as assessed by tests which measure reaction time, latency to respond, attention and speed. These conclusions are derived from group data corrected for sociodemographic variables (including socioeconomic status, educational achievement, smoking, drugs in pregnancy and obstetric medication). The results of group studies cannot be applied to individuals and tell us nothing about pathogenesis. Four distinct mechanisms by which alcohol may damage the embryo or fetus have been suggested (Table 2.3). They provide the basis for further studies both clinically and experimentally. At present it is not possible to define a safe upper limit of alcohol intake and there is no specific way of improving the development of an alcohol damaged neonate.

CHILDHOOD

Assessment

Monitoring growth and development is an invaluable means of assessing the health of a child. Retarded physical development is a non-

Table 2.3 Adverse effects of alcohol on fetal development

Time of action	Damage caused	Clinical effects
Periconceptual	Cell death Chromosomal errors	Early spontaneous abortion
Early first trimester	Cytotoxic effect	Regional agenesis Characteristic 'fetal-alcohol syndrome'
Later first trimester	Delays in neuronal migration—abnormal synapse formation	Behavioural difficulties in infancy and childhood
Post first trimester	Action on hypothalamus Poor release of GH	Growth defect

specific marker of disease. In underdeveloped countries it usually indicates primary nutritional deprivation; in the affluent world it is much more often a marker of significant chronic disease.

Height (or length), weight and skinfold thickness are the most valuable indices; head, chest and arm circumference give additional information, and in adolescents the onset and rate of development of genital and secondary sexual characteristics are also useful markers.

The processes of growth are complex and poorly understood, yet the plot of measurements obtained from a healthy child results in a remarkably smooth and reasonably predictable curve (Fig. 2.1). Growth charts are readily available (such as those from Castlemead Publications, Ware, Herts.). They are derived from data obtained from measuring single individuals at successive ages (longitudinal studies) or more commonly from averages derived from different children measured once only (cross-sectional studies). It is important to understand the difference between charts obtained by these two methods (Table 2.4). They yield different curves, especially during periods of accelerated growth, and have different uses. Cross-sectional studies are performed relatively easily and data can be obtained from a wide section of the population. The resulting charts are valuable for assessing the nutritional progress of a population and for measuring the health of cohorts of children. Longitudinal studies are rarely undertaken because it is difficult to follow a cohort of children for long enough to obtain accurate charts of growth curves. Quality control is a problem and errors of measurement are not self-cancelling. Neverthe-

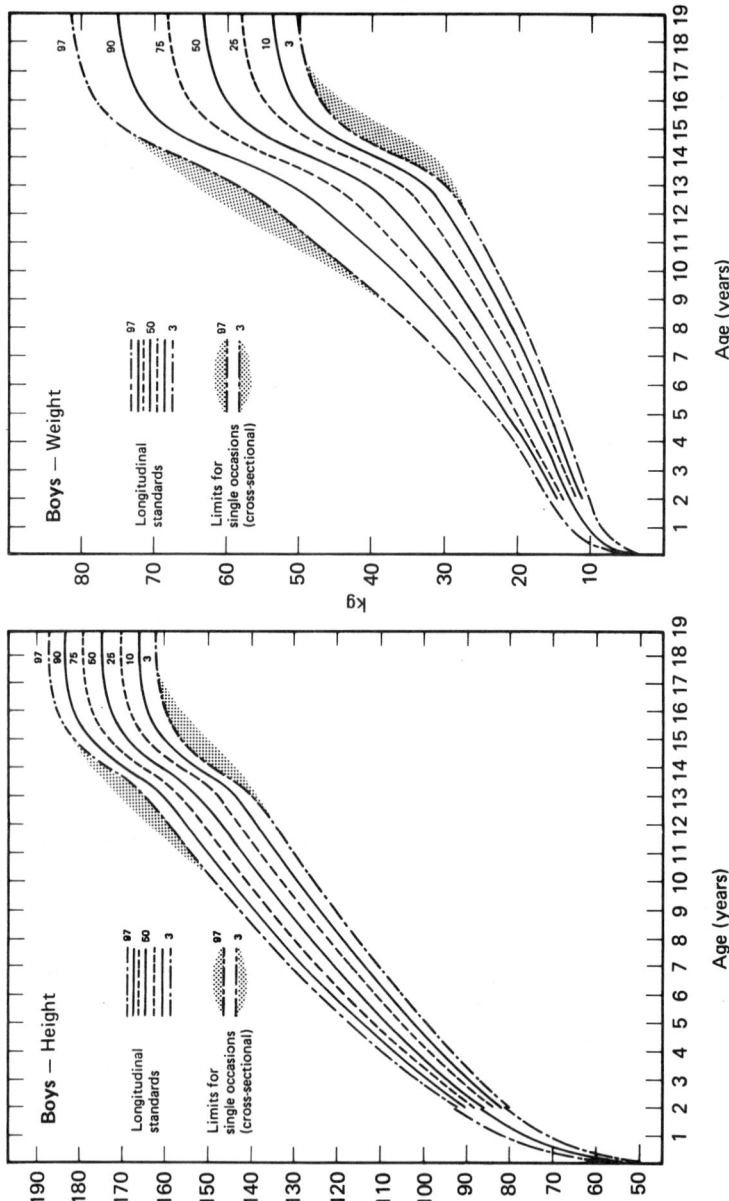

Figure 2.1 Standard growth curves for British boys. Reproduced from Tanner J. M., Whitehouse R. H. (1976). Clinical longitudinal standards for height, weight, weight velocity and stages of puberty. *Arch. Dis. Childh*; **51**: 170–9., with kind permission.

Table 2.4 Growth charts: methods of collecting data and subsequent use

Type	Method	Use
Cross-sectional	Single measurements of different children	Community studies, e.g. comparison of populations
Longitudinal		
Pure	Repeated measurements of the same group of children	
Mixed	Children of differing ages followed for as long as possible	Clinical studies
Linked	Short-term group studies (e.g. 0–5, 5–11, 10–16, 15–20 years)	

less such charts are essential for the diagnosis and treatment of individual growth disorders (particularly for the calculation of growth velocity which is so helpful in assessing treatment with growth hormone or anabolic steroids).

Modern standard growth charts are produced mathematically from an amalgam of data. The shape of the growth curves are derived from longitudinal data and absolute values from large cross-sectional surveys. Even so, such manipulations do not allow for genetic and environmental variations and one must be cautious in applying standard growth curves to the study of children in developing countries or for assessing the health of immigrant populations in a multiracial society (Table 2.5). British growth charts use the data collected by Tanner (from a cross-section of London school children in the 1950s) supplemented by the Harpenden longitudinal studies. For community studies the American National Center for Health Statistics, Health Resources Administration (NCHS) growth curves (based on cross sectional data) are the usual standard. For a description of this data see Behrman and Vaughan (1983).

Measurement techniques

Accurate measurement is of paramount importance in assessing the growing child. Routine heights and weights obtained by Clinic staff are

Table 2.5 *Differing growth characteristics of children from well-nourished populations*

Africans
  Limited data but several well-defined populations with differing growth characteristics
Americans
  Heterogenous population but:
  1. Overall the children grow faster than in the land of their forefathers
  2. Those of African origin are taller and heavier than those of European origin
Asiatics
  Considerable increase in the stature of many groups since 1950 but:
  1. Little change in the last decade
  2. Mongolian people (Chinese and Japanese) have shorter legs than Africans and Europeans and their skeletons mature earlier
Europeans
  Across the continent overall similarity in growth curves but:
  1. Urban children and those from well-off families grow faster
  2. Tallest people found in north-west Europe (Norwegians)
     Heaviest people found in south central Europe (Poles)

of no value in managing children in whom there is doubt about growth and development. The specialist clinic should have the services of a trained technician (anthropometrist) who knows how to use the instruments to achieve maximum accuracy (see Chapter 3). This is particularly important in assessing growth velocities in children receiving hormone therapy.

GROWTH AND DEVELOPMENT OF INFANTS

After birth, infants continue their prenatal growth curves. The rapid initial increase decelerates to a phase of constant velocity at about 2 years. Mid-childhood growth proceeds at a rate of rather more than 5 cm per year until the prepubertal growth spurt. Over a few months, even in completely healthy children, there may be remarkable variations in growth rate but these cancel out over a whole year. Some children grow twice as fast in summer as in winter; others (especially boys) slow down before their growth spurt.

Infant growth curves are particularly valuable in providing clinical care in underdeveloped countries. Growth charts kept in the home are useful to both the mother and the health worker/epidemiologist. Usually growth is compared against 2 lines (Fig. 2.2). The upper represents the median curve for children receiving good nutrition and good medical care; the lower gives the median growth line for village children of that country. The difference between the two lines represents the deficit due to environmental factors. Health workers are taught that their objective is to achieve growth parallel to these lines and preferably above the lower line. A sudden drop in weight is an important sign of trouble (Fig. 2.2.). An examination of the growth charts of representative children from defined areas provides a useful index of nutrition and health in those communities.

In some countries there is inadequate data regarding the growth of well infants. In such cases the fiftieth centile (boys) of a normally nourished European population provides an adequate target line. The third centile (girls) is a better lower line than the often used 80% Harvard mean (which is often given with a third line at 60% to indicate dangerous malnutrition).

Growth of the human brain

In terms of weight alone the growth spurt of the human brain starts in mid-pregnancy and begins to flatten at about 18 months of postnatal life. More than 75% of brain growth occurs after birth and cell multiplication extends well into the second year of life. On the other hand, differentiation of neuroblasts to non-dividing neurons occurs primarily from 12–18 weeks of fetal development. Glial cells continue to multiply during the rest of the period of brain growth but the increase in size is primarily due to growth of individual cells and the myelination of fibres.

Malnutrition in early pregnancy almost certainly has little or no effect on neuronal multiplication but later deprivation may affect adversely the growth of dendrites and the establishment of synaptic connections. Much has been written about the correlation between malnutrition in infancy and impaired intellectual function. Specific deficiencies of amino acids, essential fatty acids, iron, zinc or folic acid are often implicated as well as overall protein-energy malnutrition. There is little doubt that the growth of the brain may be impaired by malnutrition and that this may have important functional and behavioural consequences. Nevertheless there are many non-nutritional environmental factors which may add to or compensate for nutritional

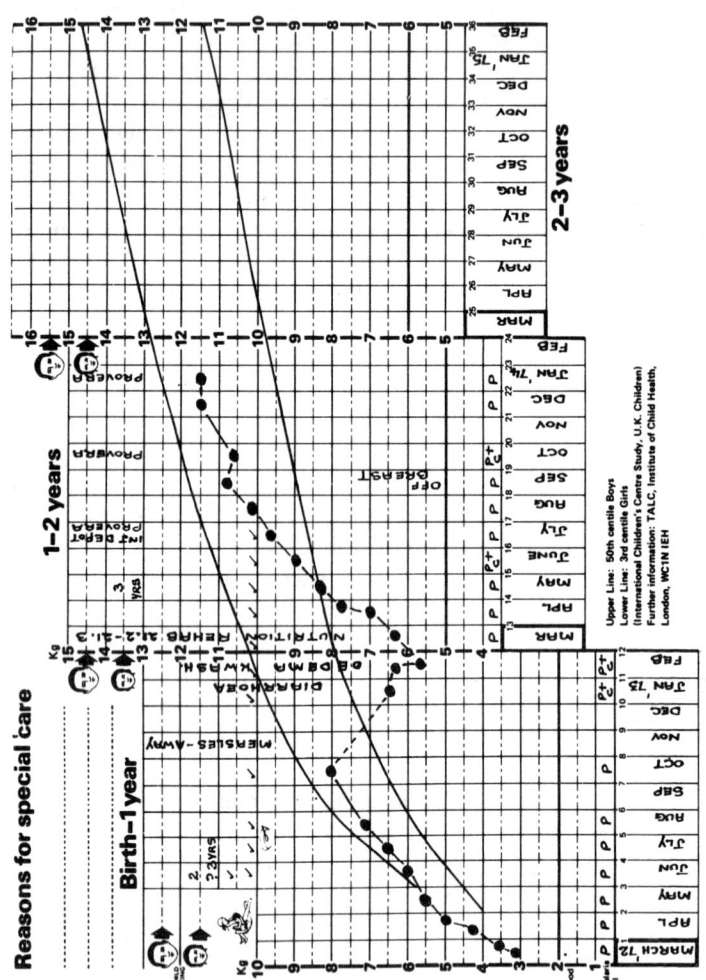

Figure 2.2 A simple growth chart for use in the Third World. Reproduced by kind permission of Dr David Morley, Professor of Tropical Child Health, University of London and Honorary Director of TALC (Teaching Aids at Low Cost), PO Box 49, St Albans, Herts.

disturbances. In the poorly fed the importance of nutrition may be no greater than any one of the many environmental components which affect intellectual function and social behaviour.

GROWTH AND DEVELOPMENT AT ADOLESCENCE

At puberty the growth spurt, the change in shape and body composition, the rapid development of the gonads, and the appearance of the secondary sexual characteristics are well defined. The hormonal control of the adolescent growth spurt differs from that of prepubertal growth. It is estimated that 30% of the variability in adult height is due to differences in the magnitude of the growth spurt. The psychological and social aspects of pubertal development are important, especially in boys. 'Early developers' are likely to dominate in physical and sexual achievements at a critical age. Clinicians need to be especially sympathetic and reassuring to 'late developers'. Adequate information about growth and its variability should be readily available to adolescents. The range of variation is considerable. Thus in affluent societies the first signs of puberty occur at about the same age in both sexes (breast buds in girls and testicular enlargement in boys) but thereafter girls mature much more rapidly and by the age of 12 or 12 and a half are 2 years ahead. The signs of pubertal development do not proceed in regular phase. A girl may reach adult physical characteristics without menstruating, a boy's genitals may develop completely in 2 years or more slowly over 5 years without relationship to the growth of pubic hair (Fig. 2.3).

OPTIMAL GROWTH AND DEVELOPMENT

In affluent societies the genes controlling growth and development may achieve their maximal expression. The effects are seen especially in the USA, Scandinavia, the Low Countries and in Australasia; but perhaps the most striking changes have occurred in Japan where there was a spectacular increase in the mean height of adults between 1950 and 1975. But is rapid growth and early physical development naturally good? For example, what is one to make of experiments which show that 'cafeteria' rats grow and mature more rapidly than their litter mates living on animal chow? The 'affluent' rats become fat and lazy

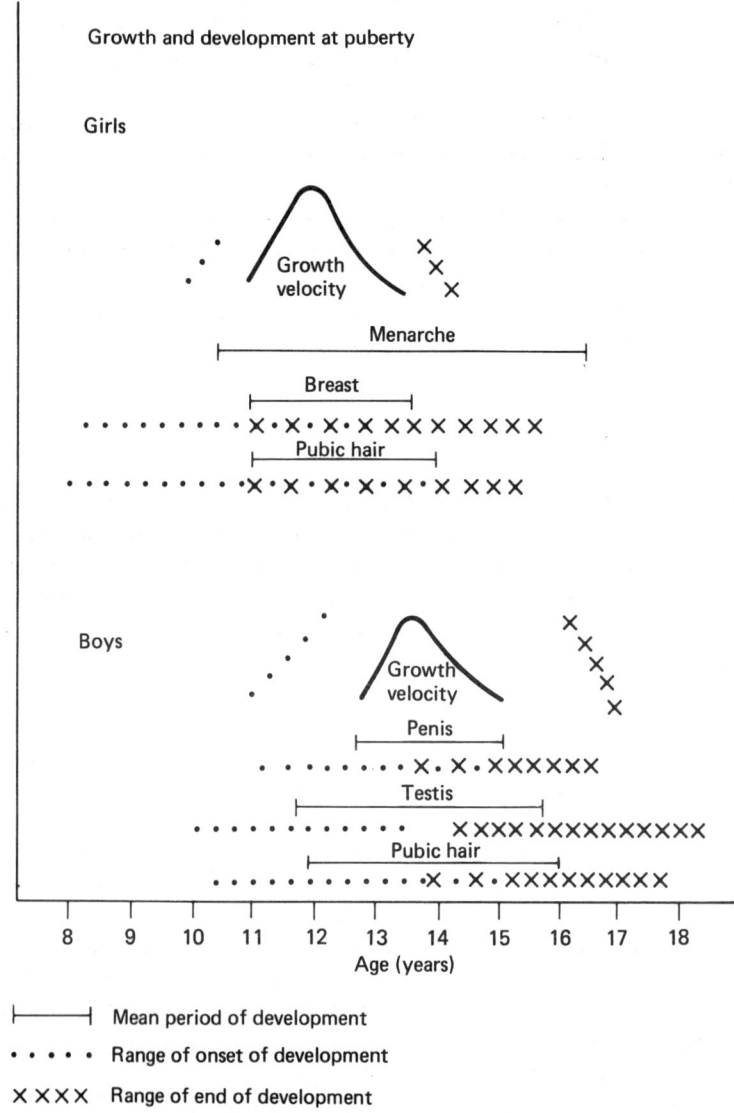

Figure 2.3 Range of age for development at puberty.

Nutrition in Growth and Development

and die earlier than those on a diet which, although well-balanced, is as monotonous as that eaten by many peasants in the Third World.

In humans equally healthy growth may be achieved more slowly with a limited intake of the energy-dense convenience foods enjoyed by children in the Western World. Growth to the maximum size permitted by the genes may not be essential for the full expression of intellectual and cultural potential. On an Earth with limited resources clear definitions of desirable energy intakes are important. Already many people in affluent countries consciously limit their energy intake in order to reduce adiposity.

The problem is complicated by genetic differences between populations. Japanese, Chinese and Indomalaysian peoples are distinctly shorter than Europeans and west Africans growing up under similar conditions (see Table 2.5). Thus growth and development must be analysed in relation to genetic potential as well as to nutrition in childhood.

Clinical implications

A century ago German paediatricians demonstrated how growth and development could be used to assess the health of the individual child. At that time, even in the middle classes, infant mortality was distressingly high. It was widely believed that factors favouring good growth also conferred increased resistance to infection (probably true although our understanding of mechanisms is extremely sketchy). With improvement in living standards clinical interest in growth waned until the 1960s when centile standards of growth suitable for clinical use first appeared. Such charts (see Fig. 2.1) are invaluable for alerting the clinician to possible latent disease and subsequently for following the response to treatment.

In affluent societies the onset of failure to thrive is often insidious. Unfortunately rather few infants have their length measured routinely during the first 2 years of life. Thus the child with a congenital disorder may not be observed to be short until its third year or even later. Charts of the growth of the constitutionally small child usually parallel the centiles of normal growth; in contrast those for the chronically sick regress although there may be periods of 'catch-up' growth coinciding with remissions of the disease process.

Delayed puberty is also a feature of some chronic illnesses. In isolation a delayed onset of puberty is difficult to interpret because of the wide range of normality (constitutional variation) (Fig. 2.3). Nevertheless delayed puberty helps children with retarded growth. Late 'catch-up' growth often leads to a more normal end-point than that suggested by plots of prepubertal height and weight.

Clinical conditions inhibiting growth and development

Children failing to grow normally require careful assessment. Sequential observations are essential and records of past measurements may be helpful in reconstructing the probable growth curves. Several possibilities must be considered in assessing the apparently healthy short child (Table 2.6). Adequate anthropometry is essential with

Table 2.6 *Causes of short stature*

1. Genetic
    Normal physiological variation
    Small stock
2. Endocrine disorders
    Low growth hormone
    Hypothyroidism
    Cushing's syndrome
3. Skeletal disorders
    Dysplastic conditions, e.g. achondroplasia
4. Failure to thrive

determination of growth velocity as the most valuable index (Fig. 2.4). It is no longer adequate practice to identify a short child (perhaps of short parents) growing on or below the fifth centile; to show normal peak values on a formal test of secretion of growth hormone and to reassure the parents that all is well. If growth velocity is outside normal limits over a whole year it is necessary to exclude latent pathology as rigorously as possible (Tables 2.6, 2.7) and if none is found to consider treatment with growth hormone.

The recognition of 'failure to thrive' opens up a wide range of possibilities (see Table 2.7). Unfortunately knowledge of pathogenic processes underlying impaired growth in chronic disease is still fragmentary (Table 2.8). Undernutrition is clearly an important factor;

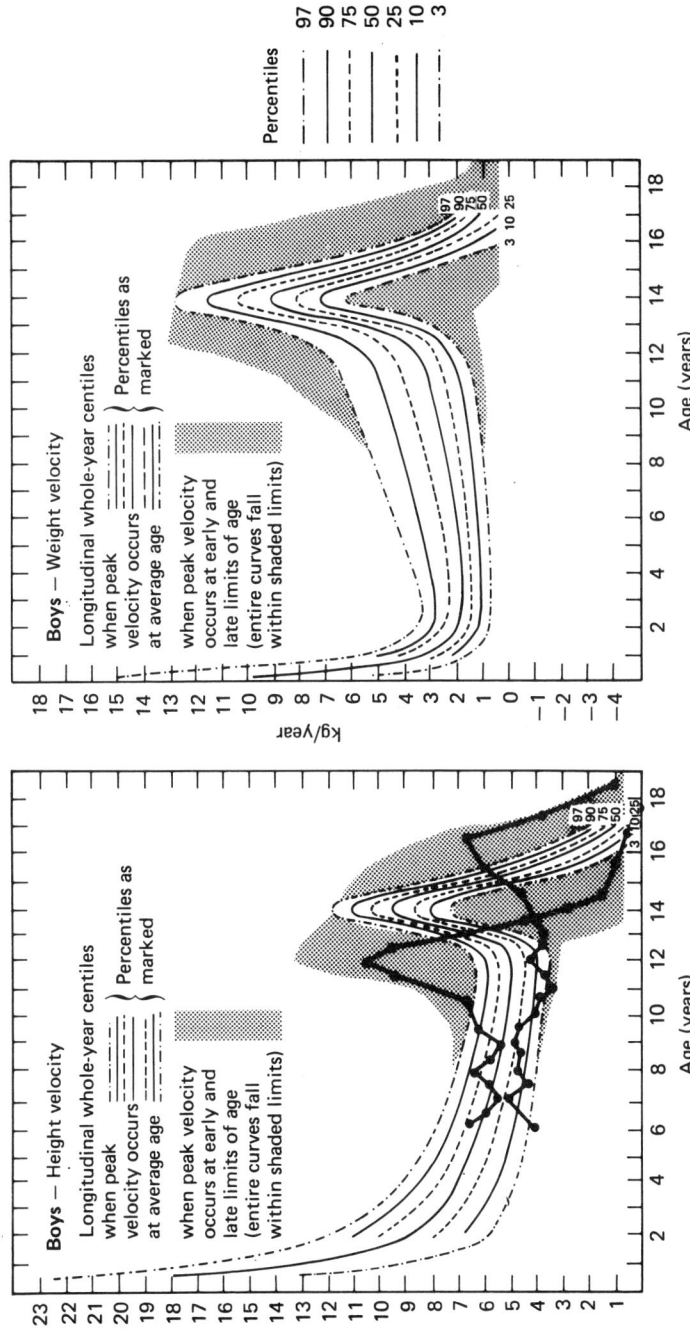

Figure 2.4 Growth velocity curves for British boys. Reproduced from Tanner J. M., Whitehouse R. H. (1976). Clinical longitudinal standards for height, weight, weight velocity and stages of puberty. *Arch. Dis. Childr*, **51**: 170–9., with kind permission.

Table 2.7 *Causes of failure to thrive*

1. Congenital systemic disorders
    Cardiac, especially cyanotic heart disease
    Renal, e.g. renal tubular acidosis
      nephrogenic diabetes insipidus
    Neurological, e.g. cerebral palsy
    Gastrointestinal, e.g. pyloric stenosis
2. Infection
    Chronic pyelonephritis
    Gastroenteritis
    Chronic chest disease, e.g. cystic fibrosis
      bronchiectasis
3. Inflammatory diseases
    Rheumatic disorders
    Inflammatory bowel disease
4. Metabolic disorders
    Diabetes mellitus
5. Malignant disease
    e.g. Wilm's tumour
6. Malabsorption
    Coeliac disease
    Pancreatic disease
    Milk protein intolerance

sick children have poor appetites. This is probably the single most important factor in their failure to grow. Dietary restrictions from other causes (unpleasant diets or food deprivation) is uncommon and severe malabsorption is easily recognized and usually not difficult to treat. Chronic undernutrition is associated with elevated levels of growth hormone (GH) but reduced values of insulin growth factor-1 (IGF1, a substance which stimulates the growth of long bones and mediates the growth-promoting action of GH). GH mobilizes fat which helps to meet the energy needs of the body. This is an important homeostatic mechanism during periods of undernutrition.

Chronic inflammation impairs growth possibly by the deviation of protein synthesis from structural proteins to those concerned with the mechanisms of defence and repair. This process is poorly understood and is difficult to disentangle from the effects of disease on appetite. Similarly chronic protein loss from the skin, the kidney or the gastrointestinal tract is often associated with impaired growth.

Table 2.8 Factors inhibiting growth and development

Primary pathology	Intra-uterine	Poor intake	Malab-sorption	Protein loss	Limited exercise	Hypoxia	Persistent inflammation	Drugs	Endocrine changes
Semi-starvation	+	+++	+ (? Gut damage)	?	Secondary	−	−	−	−
Alimentary Infant diarrhoea	−	Secondary	+	(+)	Secondary	−	?	−	−
Coeliac	−	Secondary	+++	+	−	−	−	−	GH: blunted insulin response IGF1: normal
Crohn's disease	−	Secondary	+	++	−	−	++	Steroids	IGF1: normal
Cardiac Congenital heart disease	(+)	Secondary	−	Occasional	Variable	With R–L shunts	−	−	−
Respiratory Asthma	−	?	−	−	−	(+)	−	Steroids	?Reduced nocturnal rise GH ?Effects of stress
Cystic fibrosis	(+)	+	++	−	Secondary	(+)	+	−	GH: high fasting blunted insulin response
Renal RTA	−	?	−	−	−	−	−	−	IGF1: normal Acidosis impairs bone growth
Chronic renal failure	−	++	−	Occasional	Secondary	−	(+)	−	GH: often high IGF1: reduced
Inflammatory/malignant disease	−	+	(+)	(+)	Secondary	−	++	Steroids Cytotoxics	−

+ = Conclusive evidence in favour.
(+) = Suggestive evidence in favour.
− = Evidence against.

The effects of hypoxia and of disturbances of acid–base equilibrium on growth are even less certain. The best evidence comes from animal experiments under hypoxic conditions in which reversible growth retardation can be demonstrated. Severely asthmatic children are sometimes short and the growth retardation may be correlated with the number of episodes of respiratory failure. Once again it is difficult to determine which of the disorders affecting an asthmatic are most deleterious to growth (episodes of hypoxia, increased work of breathing, disturbed sleep, episodes of infection, impaired appetite or recurrent stress).

Drugs may also inhibit growth. This is particularly true for corticosteroids and some cytotoxic agents. Corticosteroids reduce the production of pituitary growth hormone and of IGF1. They also affect protein synthesis in cartilage adversely. This is probably the most important factor and may be ameliorated by using regimens of alternate day treatment.

Primary endocrine dysfunction is probably not an important factor in growth retardation associated with chronic disease. Tests of endocrine function may give abnormal results (such as failure of GH concentrations to rise with insulin-induced hypoglycaemia; elevated resting insulin levels without hypoglycaemia; reduction of free thyroxine), but there is no clear pattern of change. Growth retardation appears to be associated with secondary changes in central hypothalamic–pituitary control. The administration of growth hormone has been shown not to improve the growth of children with disorders such as inflammatory bowel disease. In 'failure to thrive' effective treatment of the primary pathology is the only way of releasing the inhibition of growth and development (see Table 2.8).

FURTHER READING

General

Behrman R. E., Vaughan V. C. (1983). *Textbook of Pediatrics*, Chapter 2, pp. 26–35. London: Nelson.
Davis J. A., Dobbing J., eds. (1981). *Scientific Foundations of Paediatrics*. London: William Heinemann Medical Books.
Hytten F., Chamberlain G., eds. (1980). *Clinical Physiology in Obstetrics*. Oxford: Blackwell Scientific Publications.

Fetal development

Nevin N. C. (1985). The role of peri-conceptual vitamin supplementation in the prevention of neural tube defect. *Prog. Clin. Biol. Res*; **163B**: 389–96.

Smithells R. W., Sheppard S., Schorah C. J. (1976). Vitamin deficiencies and neural tube defects. *Arch. Dis. Childh*; **51**: 944–50.

Smithells R. W., Smith I. J. (1984). Alcohol and the foetus. *Arch. Dis. Childh*; **59**: 1113–14.

Infant development

Dobbing J. (1984). Infant nutrition and later development. *Nut. Rev*; **42**: 1–8.

Tanner J. M. (1986). Childhood development: physical development. *Brit. Med. Bull*; **42**: 131–8.

Chapter 3

Nutritional Assessment

BODY STRUCTURE AND FUNCTION • BODY BUILD • BODY COMPOSITION • ACTIVE TISSUE MASS • BLOOD • EXTRACELLULAR SUPPORTING TISSUES – STRUCTURAL COMPONENTS • SKIN, MUCOUS MEMBRANES AND CONNECTIVE TISSUES • MAJOR STRUCTURAL MINERALS • EXTRACELLULAR SUPPORTING TISSUE – THE FLUID COMPARTMENT • BODY CHLORIDE • VITAMINS AND TRACE ELEMENTS • PUTTING THEORY INTO PRACTICE • FURTHER READING

Sick people usually lose weight. This may be part of an adaptive response but sooner or later the signs and symptoms of malnutrition are superimposed on those of the original illness. Thus all clinicians need to be able to recognize the early indicators of significant malnutrition. Often the changes are subtle and therefore a sound knowledge of pathophysiology is necessary in order to make a valid and clinically useful assessment.

It is not enough to note that the patient is lean and to conclude that he is energy depleted, nor to record a low serum albumin and describe this as protein malnutrition, nor to treat anaemia with haematinics without determining the cause. Few symptoms or signs are diagnostic of a nutritional disorder and most laboratory results can be interpreted satisfactorily only in the light of clinical findings.

This chapter is concerned with the assessment of patients who need nutritional support to see them safely through an illness or operation. From time to time medical journals carry articles stating that 'hospitals are reservoirs of malnutrition' or that 'patients leave hospital in a poor nutritional state'. Such statements need critical examination, and clinicians need an understanding of factors affecting the measurements on which these statements are based.

Certainly, until the early 1970s nutritional support in hospitals was

Nutritional Assessment

usually limited to intravenous infusions of glucose and saline. Frequently adults would get no more than 400 kcals (1.7 MJ)/day (2 l of 5% dextrose). With prolonged illness, severe weight loss was inevitable. Today many patients receive expensive systems of nutritional support. It is important to know when and how best to provide such support and how to monitor its effect.

Unfortunately, an understanding of what can be done by nutritional means has been blurred by the lack of practical and reliable indices of nutritional status. Serum proteins, anthropometry, grip strength and a variety of 'prognostic' nutritional indices have been promoted. None has gained wide usage, primarily because it has not been possible to show that nutritional therapy alters the prognosis of patients giving abnormal results. In turn this may do no more than reflect the difficulty of undertaking clinical studies in patients with complex pathology. But there is also a failure to understand the sensitivity and specificity of tests being applied.

Experienced clinicians often rely on a simple bedside assessment to decide whether or not to give a patient artificial nutritional support. They know intuitively that nutritional assessment is not about ordering multiple investigations, demonstrating abnormal values and correcting apparent deficiencies. It is about understanding the role of nutrition in preserving organ function, in promoting pathways of intermediary metabolism appropriate to the patient's needs and in helping the body counteract pathological processes.

BODY STRUCTURE AND FUNCTION

It is necessary to have a working concept of body structure to understand what can be measured, to what degree of accuracy and with what clinical value. The body consists of an active cell mass subdivided into 2 major compartments: skeletal muscle and visceral parenchyma. It has an energy store of glycogen and fat and extracellular supporting tissue which is in part fluid and in part structural. These components cannot be quantitated accurately but estimates may be made which are useful in clinical practice (Table 3.1).

Structure, however, provides a poor index of function. Function depends not only on healthy tissues but also on an adequate supply of nutrients and specific factors (electrolytes, trace elements and vitamins) delivered by an efficient circulation. In practice nutrition is only one of

Table 3.1 Body components to be assessed in making nutritional measurements

Body structure	Value in clinical practice
1. Body build (height and weight)	Assessing growth and development in children. Monitoring effects of illness and short-term fluid balance
2. Body fat (skinfold thickness)	Assessment at nutritional extremes. Monitoring effects of artificial nutrition
3. Active cell mass	
Skeletal muscle	Muscle mass in relation to function
Viscera	Measures of visceral function, e.g. circulating proteins and immune status. (But difficult because influenced by many non-nutritional factors)
4. Extracellular supporting tissue	
Fluid (plasma, lymph, interstitial fluid)	Important day-to-day variations (water and electrolyte balance)
Structural (dermis, connective tissue, bone)	Relatively stable structures which change slowly over long periods
5. Specific substances	Needed for efficient functioning of the active cell mass
Electrolytes (including Ca, Mg, P)	Important for maintenance of *milieu intérieure*
Trace elements	Of uncertain importance in clinical practice, except for iron and possibly zinc
Vitamins	Act as enzymes and cofactors in maintaining metabolic pathways

several factors affecting organ function. Thus abnormal laboratory indices must be assessed at the bedside taking account of all processes which might alter the condition of the patient.

BODY BUILD

Height

The relationship of weight to height is a useful parameter in the assessment of nutritional status particularly in children for whom there are excellent reference data. Precise measurements are important and

Nutritional Assessment

the accuracy of instruments in every day use should be checked regularly. By convention, infants under the age of 2 years are measured supine. The clinician needs help in making this assessment. An assistant holds the infant's head firmly against the headboard; the measurer grasps the ankles, applies gentle traction and apposes the footboard to the soles of the feet in the neutral position (Fig. 3.1).

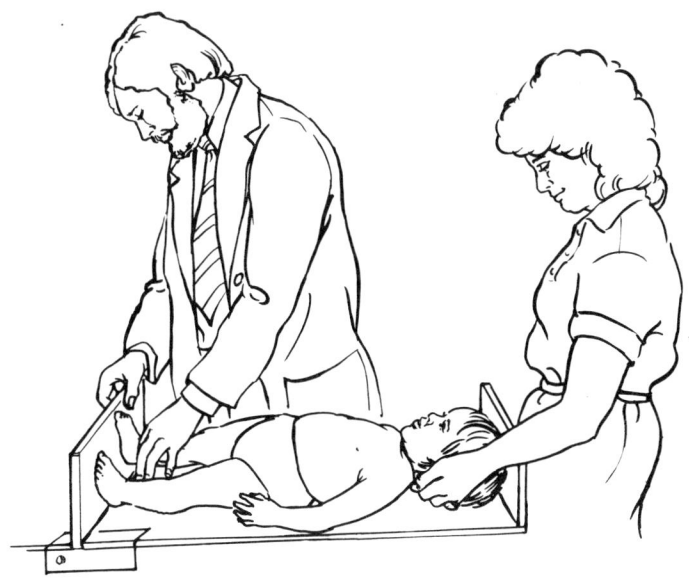

Figure 3.1 Technique for measuring the supine length of an infant.

Children over the age of 2 years are measured standing. The heels, back and occiput are aligned against a vertical surface. The trunk is stretched by applying gentle pressure on both mastoid processes and the head is settled into a neutral position, the child being instructed to look straight ahead (Fig. 3.2). A counter-balanced headboard is then brought down to rest on the vertex. A well trained observer operating under good conditions will obtain accurate and reproducible results. There is no substitute for these in the assessment of children in whom there is concern about the rate of growth (Fig. 3.3). In adults height is less important. Most people know their maximum height and this may provide useful information, especially in the elderly who have developed kyphosis of the spine.

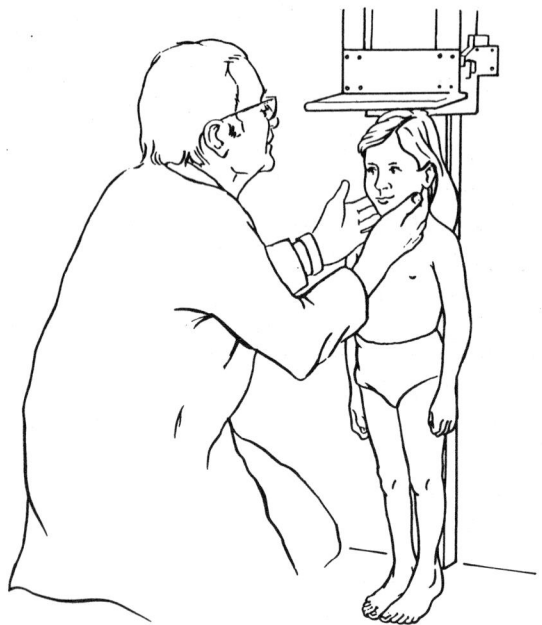

Figure 3.2 Technique for measuring standing height.

Weight

Recording the sequential weights of patients with prolonged illness provides invaluable data. It is important to remember that rapid changes in weight of several kilograms are always due to changes in hydration. It is reasonably easy to get an accurate measure of weight but instruments must be kept well calibrated. Machine error differences of 1–2 kg are not uncommon and may be sufficient to undermine the value of sequential measurements.

Height and weight of adults

Isolated weight recordings, unless extreme, are of little value for nutritional assessment. Optimal values of weight for height in adults are usually based on data obtained by the Metropolitan Life Insurance Company in the USA. It is now recognized, however, that the range of

Nutritional Assessment

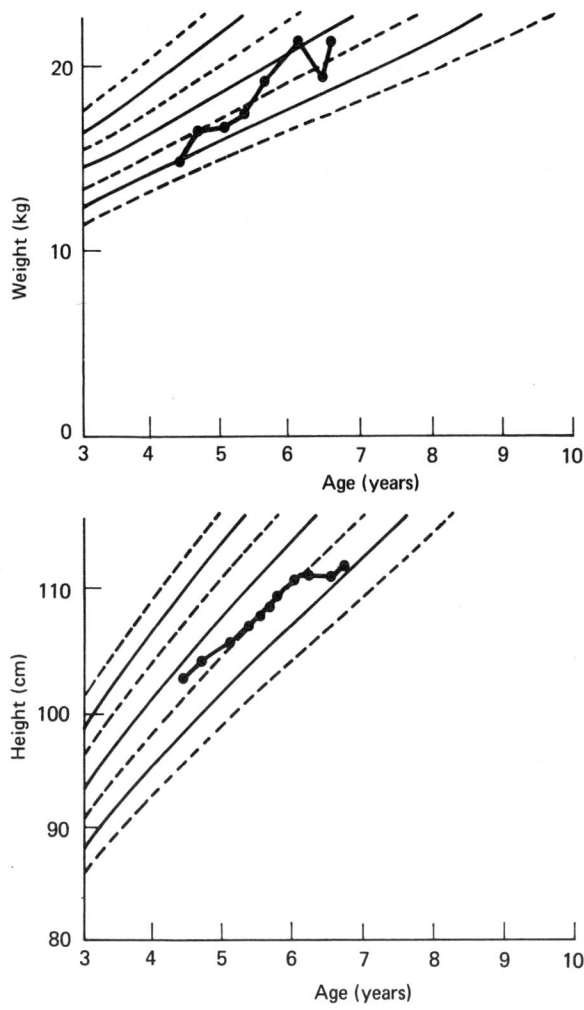

Figure 3.3 Weight and height growth curves for a girl with inflammatory bowel disease on steroids and fed parenterally for several months. Note that the weight goes from the 10th to the 50th percentile; the height drifts in the reverse direction. Steroids are stunting the growth of this child.

'healthy weight' is considerably greater than most weight tables allow (Fig. 3.4). In clinical practice sequential measurements of body weight which show systematic change are much more important than minor fluctuations.

BODY COMPOSITION

The main structural components of the body are shown in Fig. 3.5. The challenge in nutritional assessment is to find measurements which are clinically useful.

Body fat

In normal human subjects, the total mass of body fat is highly variable. Short obese females may have as much as 50% of their body weight as fat whereas well trained muscular athletes may have as little as 10%. At puberty the female gains fat relative to weight whereas the male gains skeletal muscle. Fat helps to maintain body temperature not only by providing a layer of insulation but also by modifying control mechanisms.

The body temperature of chronically sick thin patients is often 1–2°C below the normal standard. This is particularly true of the elderly. Fat may also be important in the metabolism of steroid hormones (especially oestrogens). The young woman who loses weight (such as the patient with anorexia nervosa; or the enthusiastic gymnast) often develops amenorrhoea.

Body fat is most easily estimated by measuring skinfold thickness at 4 sites (triceps, biceps, subscapular and suprailiac) (Fig. 3.6). In children the subcutaneous fat over triceps is relatively thick whereas the layer over the abdominal wall is much thinner. In adults the proportion is reversed. The topographic distribution of subcutaneous fat tends to be an individual characteristic which is, at least in part, under genetic control. Thus obese people vary in shape. In some there is a generalized increase in fat distribution; in others (especially women) there are favoured sites, especially around the pelvic girdle and on the thighs. Often it is sufficient to make a simple subjective estimate of body fat by digital pinching. A triceps skinfold thickness of less than 5 mm is usually associated with low stores of body fat. Such a patient may be at particular risk during an acute illness because of the limited

Nutritional Assessment

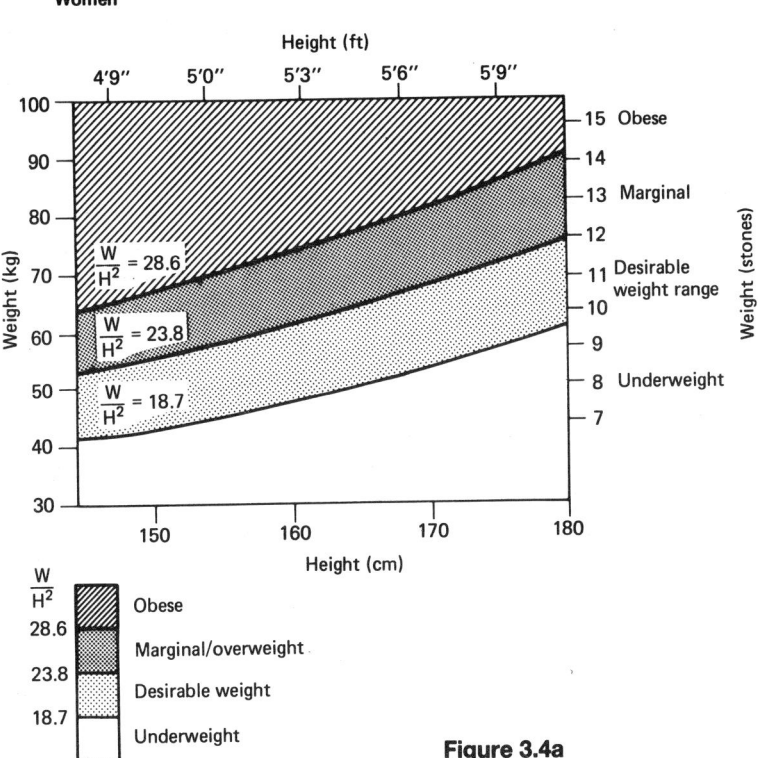

Figure 3.4a

Figure 3.4a and b Weight plotted against height for women and men. The levels for under- and overweight are arbitrary. (Fig. 3.4b see overleaf.)

stores of available energy. The correlation between energy stores and the response to stress has not been clearly defined. Nevertheless when total body fat reaches very low values physical condition deteriorates suddenly (as has been observed in people on hunger strike).

In the obese it is difficult for the clinician to assess total body fat. Skin calipers give unreliable results and some patients (especially men) store considerable fat within the abdomen. Recording changes in skinfold thickness may be useful in following the progress of sick patients requiring long-standing nutritional support.

Body protein

An effective measure of changes in total body protein and in the mass of active tissue would be extremely useful in the nutritional assessment of sick subjects. Attempts have been made using isotopes of potassium and nitrogen.

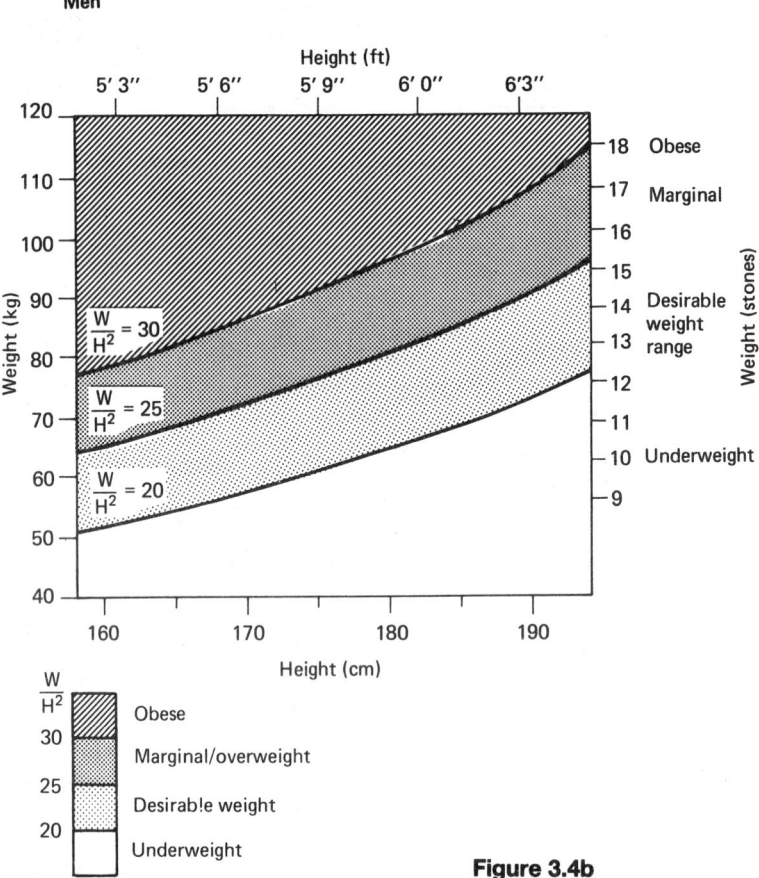

Figure 3.4b

Nutritional Assessment

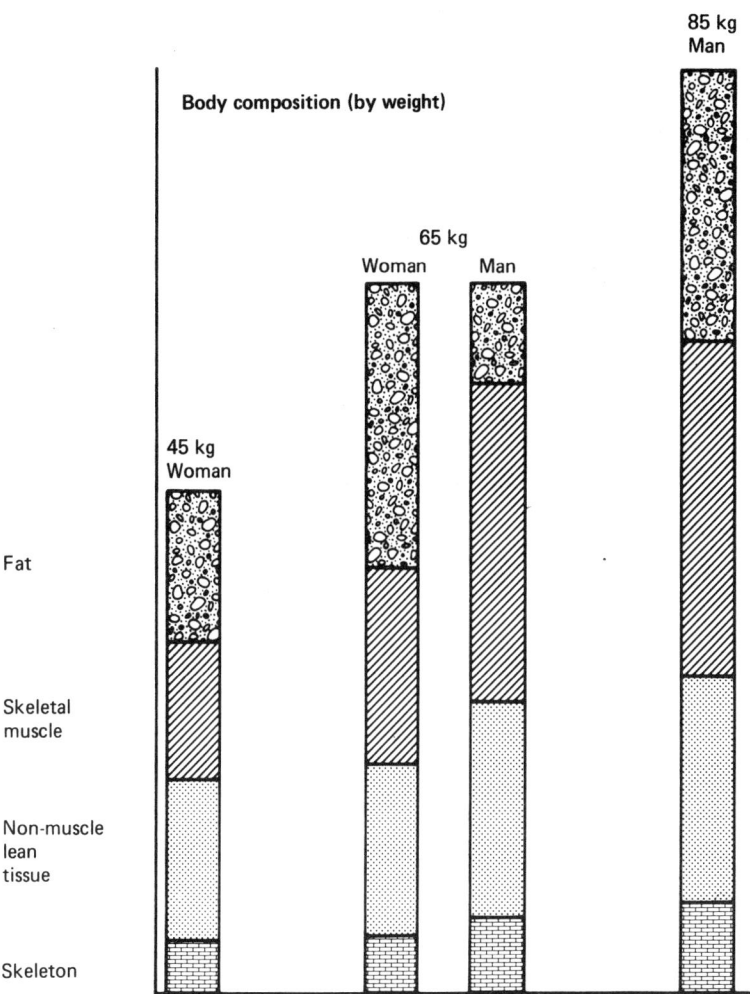

Figure 3.5 The composition of man. Note the big difference in fat and muscle in men and women of equivalent weights.

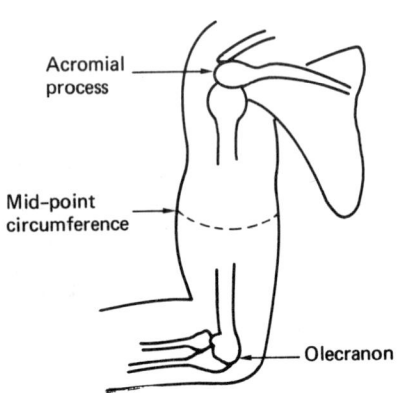 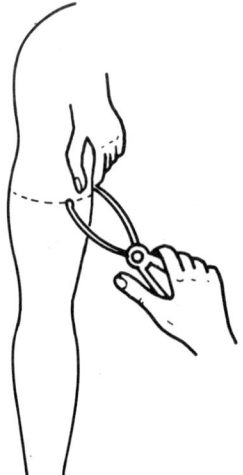

Figure 3.6 Measuring skinfold thickness. Sites:
Triceps—Over the back of the non-dominant arm at a level corresponding to a line drawn horizontally halfway between the acromial and olecranon processes. (The arm is flexed at 90% when drawing the line, then it is allowed to hang loose.)
Biceps—Anterior at the marked level with the arm resting supinated.
Subscapular—Just below the angle of the scapula in the plane of a dermatome.
Suprailiac—One centimetre above the left superior iliac crest in mid-axillary line in a horizontal plane.
Note on technique—Pull all subcutaneous tissue away gently but firmly from muscle with the middle finger and thumb of left hand. Maintain pressure and apply calipers with the right hand 1 cm away from the left hand. Maintain the pressure on the skinfold with the left hand, then release the pressure on the handle of the calipers. Read as soon as the needle has stopped moving, or within 3 s. Repeat three times and take the mean of the two closest readings. (Harpenden calipers obtainable from: Holtain Limited, Crosswell, Crymych, Dyfed.)

Body potassium

Approximately 98% of body potassium is intracellular and there is virtually none in adipocytes. It provides a means of measuring active tissue mass because potassium is readily exchangeable except for that in erythrocytes and in the skeleton. For practical purposes total body potassium is equivalent to exchangeable potassium measured using a dilution method with ^{42}K. It is also possible to estimate total body potassium by measuring the proportion of the natural isotope ^{40}K in the body. Although these methods have provided interesting data on the active tissue mass of patients in hospital, it is not a suitable method for day-to-day clinical work.

In conditions which deplete the body of potassium, such as prolonged diarrhoea, the use of diuretics and malnutrition, results are misleading. It is also difficult to make assessments of the stress of elective surgery and accidental injury in which losses of potassium and nitrogen occur in a ratio greater than those found in lean tissue. Moreover the ratio of potassium to nitrogen lost during prolonged starvation increases progressively. In extreme situations even the brain may become depleted of potassium. Conversely the deposition of glycogen in liver and skeletal muscle is associated with retention of potassium independent of changes in nitrogen balance.

Body nitrogen

Neutron activation is a valuable research tool for the measurement of body nitrogen and individual minerals, such as potassium. With neutron activation it is possible to demonstrate changes in body nitrogen over periods as short as 2 weeks. By considering concomitant changes in body potassium it is possible to show that loss of body nitrogen in wasting disorders is due more to a loss of lean tissue (of high potassium content) than of fibrous tissue (which contains little potassium). In starvation the viscera tend to be maintained at the expense of muscle. The clinician must remember that the cellular protein matrix cannot be maintained simply by providing amino acids. Cells require fluid, electrolytes, vitamins and essential fatty acids, an effective stimulus and an appropriate source of energy in order to put the building blocks together.

Nitrogen (protein) balance

In practice it may be possible to do no more than measure *changes* in the protein content of the active cell mass. This can be estimated by a simplified study of nitrogen balance. Intake is measured by weighing the food ingested and output estimated from the equation:

Nitrogen losses = Urinary nitrogen + faecal nitrogen
(other losses are negligible unless the patient has a fistula)

Urinary nitrogen (g) = Urine urea (g) $\times \dfrac{28}{60} \times \dfrac{6}{5}$

(because nitrogen makes up 28 parts of the molecular weight of urea (60) and 20% is added for non-urea nitrogen)

or Urine urea (mmol) $\times$ 0.028 $\times$ 1.2

Faecal nitrogen = 1–2 g/day (usual to allow 2 g total to cover faecal and skin losses)

These estimates assume a steady state. Additional factors must be added for proteinuria and losses via fistulae. A correction must also be made for changes in circulating blood urea:

Change in nitrogen (g) = Change in blood urea (mmol/l) $\times$ 3/5 body weight (kg) $\times$ 0.028
(Body water = 60% body weight)

Nitrogen balance may be used for the evaluation of nutritional requirements. Patients in whom nitrogen balances are negative require careful assessment. Are they intensely catabolic? Are they getting sufficient nitrogen? Are they deficient of key cell constituents, such as potassium or magnesium? For short periods after severe trauma, it is not possible to prevent some protein wasting. Under such circumstances the giving of very large amounts of nitrogen (usually as amino acids intravenously) is not only ineffective but may be harmful.

ACTIVE TISSUE MASS

The active tissue mass comprises two major elements: skeletal muscle and the body viscera.

Skeletal muscle

Skeletal muscle is the largest single body tissue. Unfortunately, without exercise, skeletal muscle wastes so measurement of size is not necessarily a good nutritional index. A simple measure of muscle bulk (Table 3.2) may be helpful in assessing the patient who has lost considerable

Table 3.2 *Measurement of muscle mass* (see Heymsfield et al., 1982)

1. *Anthropometry*
Muscle mass (kg) = Height (cm) × (0.0264 + 0.0029 × CMA) where CMA = the corrected muscle area for the upper arm
Uncorrected muscle area (UMA) = $(C-\pi T)^2/4\pi$ cm^2 where C = limb circumference (cm); T = skinfold thickness (cm)
Corrected muscle area (CMA) takes account of enclosed bone and soft tissue
For men CMA = (UMA−10) cm^2
For women CMA = (UMA−6.5) cm^2

2. *Creatinine excretion*
In healthy subjects on a low animal fat diet, the excretion of creatinine is proportional to the mass of skeletal muscle:

Total muscle mass (kg) = 24 h excretion creatinine (g) × 18
(mmol) × 2

The conversion factor is only approximate; the formula does not hold true for sick patients, and it is difficult to get an accurate and reproducible assessment of creatinine excretion

3. *Comparative data*
   (a) Normal values for upper arm muscle area (uncorrected UMA)

Age	Centile:	Female 5	50	95	Centile:	Male 5	50	95
19–24.9		25.4	34.1	49.4		45.1	59.1	82.0
25–34.9		26.6	35.7	55.4		46.9	62.1	84.4
35–44.9		27.5	37.8	58.8		48.4	64.9	84.9
45–54.9		27.8	38.6	59.6		45.5	63.0	84.6
55–64.9		27.8	40.5	62.5		44.2	61.4	81.5
65–74.9		27.4	40.2	62.1		39.7	57.2	74.5

   (b) Height, weight and creatinine excretion

Height (H) cm	Acceptable weight (unclothed) kg		Creatinine (C) g excretion in 24 h		C/H Index	
	Female	Male	Female	Male	Female	Male
150	39–56		0.85		0.57	
155	42–60		0.90		0.58	
160	44–62	46–66	0.95	1.32	0.59	0.82
165	46–65	49–70	1.00	1.38	0.61	0.83
170	48–68	52–74	1.07	1.46	0.63	0.86
175	51–72	55–78	1.14	1.55	0.64	0.88
180	53–75	58–83	1.20	1.64	0.66	0.91
185		62–88		1.73		0.94
190		65–92		1.82		0.96

Heymsfield S. B., McManus C., Smith J., Stevens V., Nixon D. W. (1982). Anthropometric measurement of muscle mass: revised equations for calculating bone-free arm muscle area. *Amer. J. Clin. Nut.*; **38**: 680–90.

weight (has he lost muscle as well as fat?) and the patient who is weak (see Table 3.4). There are no simple methods for the accurate measurement of total body muscle mass. The anthropometric method makes use of the formula devised by Heymsfield and his coworkers. (Heymsfield *et al.*, 1982). The creatinine method (Table 3.2) assumes an excretion of 23 mg creatinine per kilogram of muscle mass for males and 18 mg/kg for females. The values diminish with age. Some workers recommend a correction for height and use the creatinine : height ratio. The method is rarely used in clinical practice. Nevertheless in following the progress of patients a crude measure of muscle mass (e.g. UMA) may be helpful (see Table 5.8).

Muscle mass

Muscle mass varies enormously between normal individuals. On graphs of muscle area there is a 2- to 3-fold difference between the 5th and 95th centiles (Fig. 3.7). Moreover, immobilization, denervation, or myopathic disorders may be associated with considerable muscle wasting in the presence of adequate nutrition. Thus most experienced clinicians pay little attention to absolute measurements of muscle mass. They may note generalized wasting and use this as a marker of the need for supplementary feeding.

Muscle function

Muscle strength is markedly reduced in the severely malnourished. Recently clinicians have been assessing simple methods of measurement (Table 3.3) which might be of value in patient management. In normal subjects muscle strength correlates well with muscle mass but in sick patients weakness may be due to many factors, mostly non-nutritional. Weakness of grip strength may be used to predict the likelihood of postoperative morbidity but usually it is not possible to correct such weakness solely by nutritional means.

Muscle biopsy

Muscle biopsy is not often required for diagnostic purposes. Occasionally it may be of value in helping to determine the cause of muscle weakness without wasting. It is important to remember the causes of myopathy (Table 3.4).

Nutritional Assessment

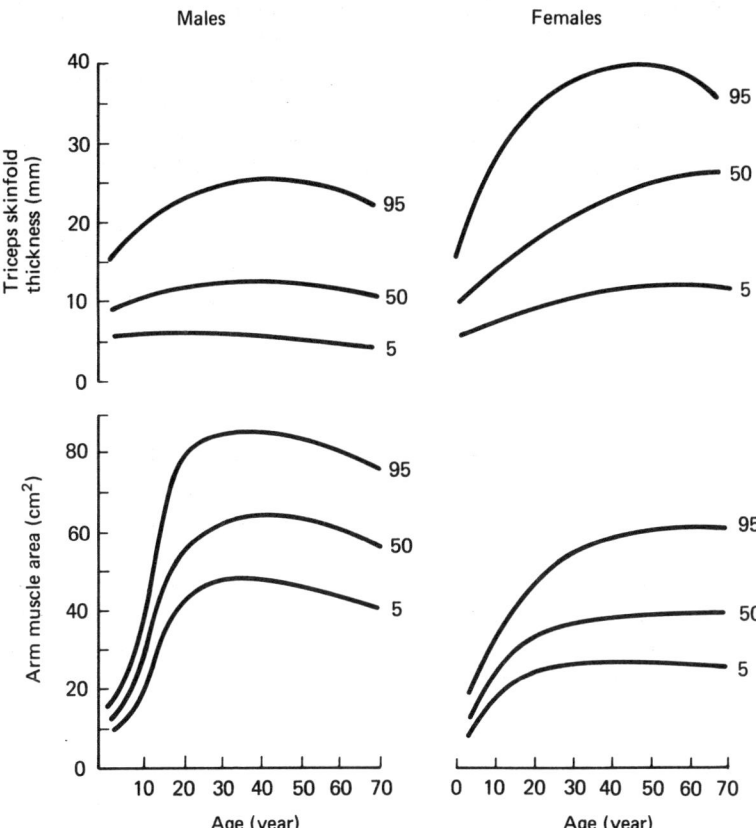

Figure 3.7 Percentile curves for triceps skinfold thickness and estimated muscle area derived from an analysis of US data obtained in Health and Nutrition Survey. (Frisancho A. R. (1984). New standards of weight and body composition by frame size and height for the assessment of nutritional status of adults and of the elderly. *Amer. J. Clin. Nut*; **40**: 808–19. Also Frisancho A. R. (1981). New norms of upper limb fat and muscle areas for assessment of nutritional status. *Amer. J. Clin. Nut*; **34**: 2540–5.)

The viscera

Extreme deficiencies of specific nutrients may cause well-characterized disorders of certain viscera (Table 3.5). In dealing with the effects of

Table 3.3 *Measurement of muscle function*

Movement	Muscles involved	Method
Thumb adduction	Adductor pollicis	Electrical stimulation[1]
Grip	Long flexors	Grip strength[2]
Knee extension	Quadriceps, rectus, tensors fasciae	Special chair[3]

1. Russell D. McR., Prendergast P. J., Darby P. L., *et al.* (1983). Skeletal muscle function during hypocaloric diet and fasting: a comparison with standard nutritional assessment parameters. *Amer. J. Clin. Nut.*; **37**: 133–8.
2. Karran S. (1982). Who needs nutritional support? In *Surgical Review*, 3rd edn. (Lumley S. J. P., Craven J. L., eds.) pp. 25–62. London: Pitman.
3. Maxwell J. D., Hodt P., Taylor W. H. (1984). Portable chair for testing isometric muscle strength. *Lancet* **1**: 18–19.

Table 3.4 *Common causes of proximal myopathy*

Endocrine
    Cushing's syndrome
    Corticosteroid therapy
    Thyrotoxicosis
Carcinoma
    Especially lung, breast, prostrate, gastrointestinal tract
Deficiency
    Vitamin D
Alcohol

low-grade generalized malnutrition, however, disturbances of visceral function are difficult to assess.

Visceral function

Malnutrition may adversely affect five major body functions: those

Table 3.5 Visceral disorders as a result of nutrient deficiencies

Nutrient deficiency	Visceral disorder
Protein (Energy intake maintained)	Fatty liver, hypoproteinaemia, often multiorgan failure (e.g. pancreas, small gut)
Mineral	
Iron	Microcytic hypochromic anaemia
B12/Folate	Megaloblastic anaemia
Zinc	Acrodermatitis
Selenium	Cardiomyopathy
Iodine	Thyroid deficiency
Potassium	Skeletal muscle weakness
Phosphate	Skeletal muscle weakness
Vitamins	
A	Xerophthalmia
B	Neurological structures damaged (peripheral neuropathy, encephalopathy)
K	Coagulation factors damaged

concerned with physical activity, reproductive competence, cognitive ability, social/behavioural performance and the response to challenge by pathological agents. These facets of body function are difficult to measure in a clinical setting. Nevertheless the skilled clinician will not have great difficulty in considering a nutritional disorder, such as coeliac disease, when assessing a physically poorly developed child with delayed puberty, who is not doing well at school and who appears to be susceptible to infection.

In clinical practice three aspects of visceral function have been used as markers of nutritional status: the ability of the liver to produce 'export' proteins, the response of the immune system to challenge and the assessment of pathways of intermediate metabolism. As with most other nutritional measurements interpreting the results is not easy.

Hepatic secretory proteins. Most circulating proteins are produced by the liver, and their concentrations in the circulation can be measured quite readily. As a result they have been used extensively and often quite uncritically in the assessment of nutritional status. Serum albumin is usually regarded as a key marker of protein-energy malnutrition but its concentration reflects not only synthesis rate but also losses of protein from the body, tissue catabolism and distribution of albumin in body pools (Fig. 3.8).

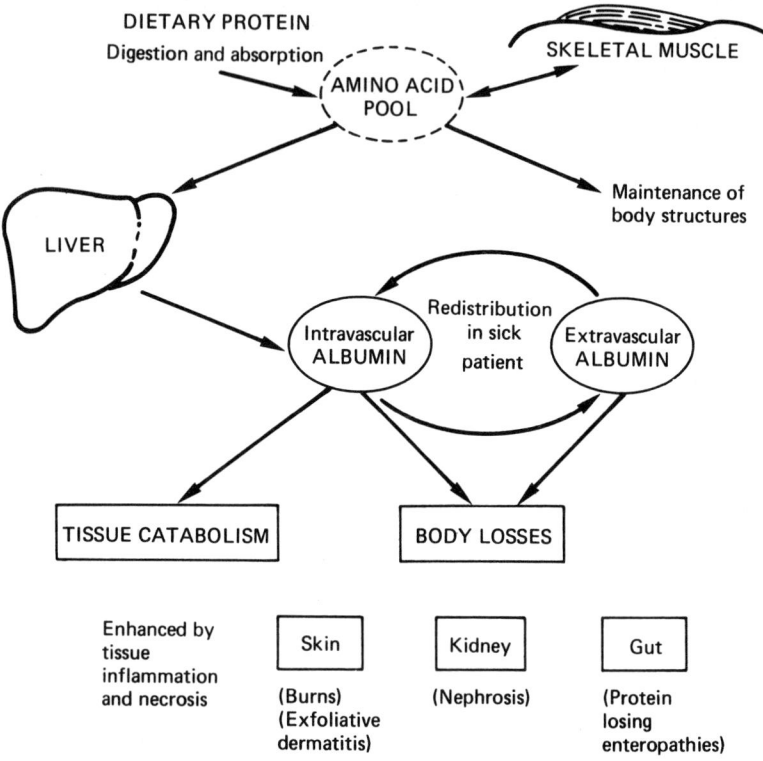

Figure 3.8 Factors influencing the concentration of circulating albumin.

The total albumin mass is about 300 g, more than half of which is extravascular. Passage of albumin from the intravascular space (transcapillary escape) occurs continuously at a rate of about 5%/h. Escaped albumin is returned to the circulation by the lymphatics. In disease, the proportion of albumin in intravascular and extravascular pools varies. In fact in contrast to injury and inflammation, starvation is usually associated with a preferential preservation of the intravascular albumin mass. Thus the concentration of plasma albumin is maintained in obese patients losing weight and in patients with anorexia nervosa. The normal catabolism of albumin gives a half-life of 12–20 days, but this is readily enhanced by inflammatory disorders. Likewise, the synthesis rate is altered by non-nutritional factors such as infection. Thus the concentration of circulating albumin is readily affected by clinical disorders most of which are not nutritionally determined.

The half-life of albumin is too long for the recognition of a rapid response and thus it is reasonable to consider changes in other proteins with shorter half-lives, e.g. transferrin (5 days) pre-albumin (2 days) and retinal-binding protein (10 h). Once again, however, the clinician must take into account possible confounding factors (Table 3.6).

Table 3.6 *Factors affecting the concentration of circulating proteins*

Protein	Increased concentrations	Decreased concentrations
All proteins	Dehydration	Overhydration Nephrotic syndrome Protein-losing enteropathy
Albumin		Injury/inflammation Cirrhosis
Pre-albumin		Acute starvation Injury/inflammation Liver disease
Transferrin	Iron deficiency Pregnancy (Oestrogens)	As for pre-albumin
Retinol binding protein	Renal insufficiency (Corticosteroids)	As for pre-albumin Vitamin A deficiency Zinc deficiency
Acute phase proteins		
Haptoglobin	Injury/inflammation	Haemolysis Ineffective erythropoiesis
α_1-Antitrypsin	Injury/inflammation (but variable)	
Orosomucoid	Injury/inflammation Renal insufficiency	

Curiously, the plasma concentration of a short half-life protein in a normal individual may fall quite rapidly over a few days of dietary deprivation and yet is often normal or near-normal in a patient with well-established malnutrition.

The immune response. The immune response is blunted in severely malnourished subjects. Although the concentration of immunoglobulins is well maintained, there is a decrease in secretion of IgA into the gut and bronchi, and cell-mediated immunity may be markedly impaired. The absolute count of circulating lymphocytes is often low (less than $1500/mm^3$). Although the specificity of this finding is uncertain, it is a simple laboratory measurement which may be of some value in assessing the patient's overall response to a serious pathological process.

Delayed cutaneous hypersensitivity responses to common recall antigens have been used as markers of immune status associated with malnutrition. Unfortunately such tests are also adversely affected by increasing age, body trauma, infection and malignancy. Moreover, skin-prick tests are often not readily reproducible. In the UK few clinicians use skin testing routinely as a marker of nutritional depletion.

Tests of pathways of intermediary metabolism. Malnutrition may interfere with enzyme systems thereby affecting metabolic pathways adversely (Table 3.7). These are not used routinely.

Table 3.7 In vivo *tests of intermediate metabolism*

Substrate	Metabolite	Deficiency
Histidine	Urinary urocanic acid	Protein
	Urinary formimino-glutamic acid	Folic acid
Tryptophan	Urinary xanthurenic acid	Pyridoxine
Leucine	Urinary 3HO-valeric acid	Biotin
Glucose	Blood lactate/pyruvate	Thiamin

BLOOD

The formed elements in blood make up one of the body's vital organs. A blood count and the examination of a blood film are important in nutritional assessment. As with other components of the active tissue mass, however, these laboratory measurements are markedly affected by non-nutritional factors, especially infection, inflammatory conditions, blood loss and changes in body hydration.

Haematological indices

Haemoglobin, mean corpuscular volume (MCV), mean corpuscular haemoglobin concentration (MCHC), red cell morphology, white cell count and morphology and platelet count, should all be assessed (Table 3.8). They provide useful indicators to possible deficiencies of iron, vitamin B12, folic acid, and the rare anaemias of scurvy and of pyridoxine deficiency.

Table 3.8 Haematological indices: alterations observed with deficiencies of iron, folic acid or vitamin B12

Index	Normal values	Iron deficency	B12/Folate deficiency
Red cell count	$5.5 \pm 1.0 \times 10/1$ (men) $4.8 \pm 1.0 \times 10/1$ (women)	Often maintained	Falls
Haemoglobin (Hb)	15.5 ± 2.5 g/dl (men) 14.0 ± 2.5 g/dl (women)	Falls but with early deficiency may be within normal limits	
Packed cell volume (PCV)	0.47 ± 0.07 (men) 0.42 ± 0.05 (women)	Falls	Falls
Mean cell volume (MCV)	77–95 fl	Decreases (50–80)	Increases (100–140)
Mean corpuscular haemoglobin (MCH)	27–32 pg	<27	33–38
Mean corpuscular Hb concentration (MCHC = Hb/PCV)	31–35 g/dl	Insensitive	
White cell count	$(4-11) \times 10/l$	Normal	Falls
Platelet count	$(150-400) \times 10/l$	Raised if bleeding	May fall (Occasionally very low)

Bone marrow

Examination of the bone marrow is necessary to confirm a suspected megaloblastosis which signifies lack of vitamin B12 or folic acid. It also provides a valuable method of assessing iron stores and the sideroblastic changes of pyridoxine deficiency. Severe iron deficiency may mask the megaloblastic changes of vitamin B12 or folic acid deficiency although giant metamyelocytes usually persist among the white cell precursors.

Haematinics

Iron

Circulating concentrations of iron and iron-binding capacity are too readily altered by the systemic effects of inflammatory and neoplastic disease to provide reliable indices of iron status. Ferritin may prove to be a better marker, but concentrations of this protein rise in inflammatory conditions.

Folic acid

Serum values of folic acid decline rapidly in subjects eating poorly. Thus serum folate is a poor indicator of body stores. These are best assessed by measuring the concentration of folate in red cells.

In acutely sick patients, especially those requiring intensive care, the body may not be able to mobilize body stores of folate. In this situation red cell morphology may remain normal yet the patient can develop a profound leukopenia and thrombocytopenia. Often it is not possible to confirm the diagnosis with certainty but there should be a rapid response to treatment with folic acid. Some authorities prefer to use folinic acid to overcome a possible block in folate metabolism.

Vitamin B12

In contrast to folic acid the concentration of vitamin B12 in the plasma gives a reasonably sensitive index of body stores, although in hepatic disease or severe malnutrition circulating levels may be affected by an increase in the transport protein transcobalamin II. In practice serum levels of less than 100 ng/ml are virtually diagnostic of vitamin B12 deficiency. Values of between 100 and 180 ng/ml are difficult to interpret, especially in patients with serious pathology and in those taking drugs such as anticonvulsants.

EXTRACELLULAR SUPPORTING TISSUES – STRUCTURAL COMPONENTS

Body structural tissues change relatively slowly with pathological processes, although calcium may be lost from bone at quite an alarming rate with immobility or as a result of the long-continued use of drugs, such as corticosteroids or heparin.

Bone

Bone mineral in healthy people depends on genetic, developmental and environmental factors. The role of nutrition during development is not clearly established. There are few data on bone density during childhood and these are not used in clinical assessment except in relationship to rickets. In contrast bone wasting disorders in the adult are of considerable clinical importance. Osteoporosis and osteomalacia (equivalent to rickets in childhood) are the two disorders of bone structure which may be caused by inadequate nutrition.

Osteoporosis

It is still not clear whether osteoporosis should be regarded as a disorder of protein matrix or simply the result of negative calcium balance, small in quantity, but continued over a long time. Almost certainly a number of mechanisms are involved. Osteoporosis is frequently regarded as a normal manifestation of ageing. Bone loss in old age, however, has not been conclusively related to calcium intake in adult life even though the amount of bone present in later years does appear to be directly related to the skeletal mass at maturity.

Diagnosis, during the early stages of accelerated calcium loss, is difficult. Bone mass may be assessed by a variety of scanning techniques: densitometry, radiogravimetry, photon beam scanning and computerized tomography. These procedures yield interesting data but are rarely used in routine practice.

Characteristically, the axial skeleton is more subject to osteoporotic processes than the long bones. Radiographs of the spine provide the most practical method of assessing bone density. In osteoporosis there is thinning of cortical bone with an overall loss of bone contrast. The distance between normally mineralized but thin trabeculae increases, and there is concomitant loss of transverse trabeculae (hence 'osteoporosis') (Fig. 3.9). Crush fractures of the spine with collapse of vertebral endplates and anterior wedging of the bodies are characteristic in the later stages but these findings are not specific (multiple myeloma, for example, may present in the same way).

Rickets and osteomalacia

Rickets in children and osteomalacia in adults are caused primarily by a deficiency of vitamin D, although there may be contributory factors such as the effects of long-continued acidosis on calcium absorption and metabolism, or the ingestion of cereal products containing excessive amounts of phytate.

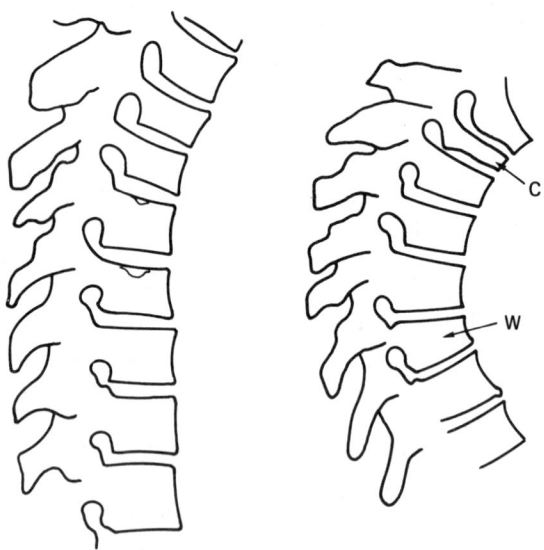

Figure 3.9 Characteristic wedging (W) and crushing (C) of vertebrae in the osteoporotic spine.

Vitamin D is misnamed. It should be regarded as a hormone, cholecalciferol, rather than as an essential nutrient. There is little vitamin D in the British diet and what there is behaves as a supplement to that produced in the skin by irradiation with ultraviolet light. The requirements for vitamin D are uncertain but are of the order of 10–20 µg (400–800 IU)/day. In hospital practice low grade osteomalacia is probably quite common, particularly in the elderly and in patients with long-standing gastrointestinal disorders.

Biochemical and radiological investigation are used most often in trying to establish a diagnosis of osteomalacia, although modern techniques of radioisotope scanning using labelled diphosphonates are gaining favour. In the malacic subject plasma calcium (corrected for albumin) and phosphate (measured in blood taken fasting) both tend to fall and the serum alkaline phosphatase rises. Unfortunately any or all of these variables may remain normal in vitamin D-deficient patients even in the presence of histologically-proven osteomalacia. Circulating levels of 25 - hydroxycholecalciferol (25HOCC) give a useful measure of vitamin D status even though there is a seasonal variation. The normal range varies somewhat from centre to centre. In general, however, values below 8 nmol/l are usually associated with malacic bones whereas intermediate values (8–16 nmol/l) are less helpful in making a diagnosis. Parathormone (PTH) increases in most subjects with osteomalacia but is not a sensitive index and may remain unchanged if there is concomitant magnesium deficiency.

In suspected cases of osteomalacia (rickets) isotope scanning is a sensitive screening test. Enhanced uptake of diphosphonate, however, is not specific for osteomalacia. For example, it is also found in hyperparathyroidism and other conditions with a generalized increase in bone turnover (e.g. 'active osteoporosis'). Looser's zones (see below) are readily visualized and, if present, are diagnostic of the malacic process.

Radiology is less sensitive than isotope scanning but is helpful in elucidating combined pathology (e.g. Paget's disease in a malacic subject). The hands, thorax and pelvis should be screened. Looser's zones (especially on the medial edges of the scapulae, the pelvic rami and the femoral necks), the subperiosteal erosions of secondary hyperparathyroidism (especially well seen in the phalanges) and the characteristic metaphyseal changes of rickets may provide conclusive evidence of vitamin D deficient bone disease (Fig. 3.10). More often the radiographs are normal or show no more than non-specific demineralization perhaps because of associated osteoporosis.

Quantitative histology of biopsies taken from the iliac crest provides the best direct evidence of the failure of calcification of newly-formed osteoid which is the hallmark of osteomalacia (Fig. 3.11).

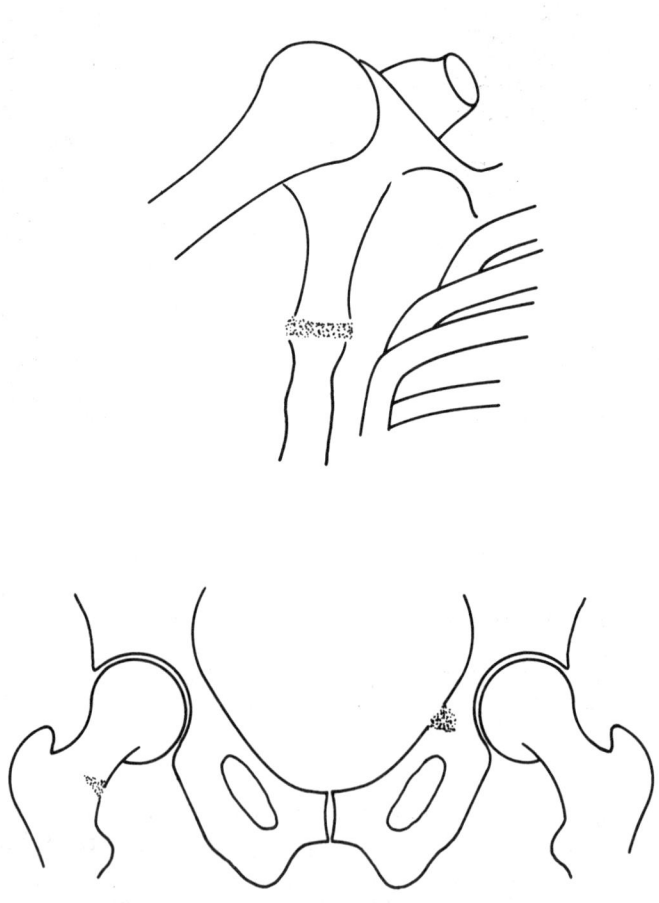

Figure 3.10 Common sites for Looser's zones: lateral edge of scapula, medial edge of neck of femur, superior public ramus. The decalcification of cortical bone is pathognomic of osteomalacia.

Nutritional Assessment

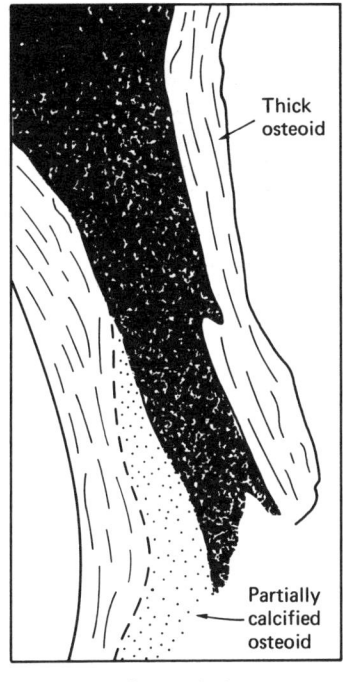
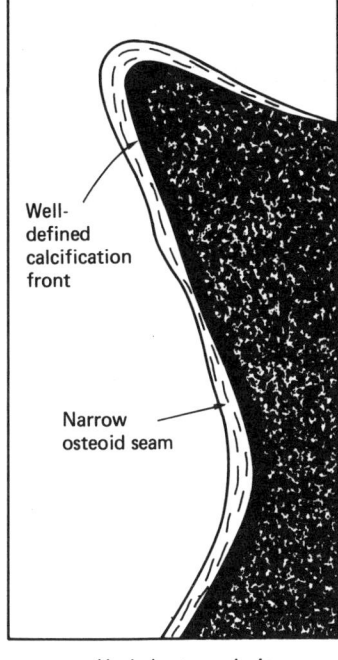

Osteomalacia

Histology of osteomalacic bone shows
  Wide osteoid seams
  Patchy calcified osteoid
  Poorly defined calcification front

Healed osteomalacia

Histology of normal bone shows
  Narrow osteoid seams
  Well-defined calcification front

Figure 3.11 Histological features of osteomalacic bone. Osteoid seams are wide, newly formed osteoid shows only patchy calcification and the calcification point is poorly defined. These findings are contrasted with histological findings after the administration of vitamin D.

In practice suspected vitamin D deficiency is often treated without recourse to biopsy of bone. The response to treatment should be monitored carefully because overdosing may lead to hypercalcaemia and its attendant disorders. The response to 1 mg cholecalciferol given intravenously has been used as a diagnostic test. In a patient with osteomalacia it leads to a prompt rise in fasting serum phosphate and a rather slower increase in serum calcium. The serum alkaline phosphatase increases temporarily and then may take several weeks to return to normal. In general, however, parenteral milligram doses of calciferol are unnecessary in the management of patients with nutritional vitamin D deficiency. Usually it is sufficient to give 25–50 µg/day orally (see p. 95). If available graded doses of ultraviolet light (most easily obtained through the physiotherapy department) also provide a simple and safe method of treating nutritional vitamin D deficiency. In a case in which the diagnosis of osteomalacia is in doubt repeated measurements of the retention of low doses of diphosphonate given at intervals of 3–6 months provides a useful index of the effects of therapy.

SKIN, MUCOUS MEMBRANES AND CONNECTIVE TISSUES

The skin, hair and nails, and mucous membranes may provide helpful clues in assessing nutritional status (Table 3.9). In clinical practice,

Table 3.9 Physical signs of nutritional deficiency as seen on examination of the integument

Sign	Possible nutrient deficiency
Easy bruising	Vitamin C (scurvy—positive Hess test) Vitamin K
Dry scaly skin	Usually non-specific (but occurs with essential fatty acid deficiency)
Peristomal and acral bullous/pustular eruption	Zinc
Sparse depigmented hair	Long-standing malnutrition (especially Kwashiorkor)
Koilonychia	Iron (but may be genetic)
Leuconychia	Protein (but any serious illness may impair synthesis of keratin)
Angular stomatitis Naso-labial seborrhoea	? Vitamin B but common especially in the elderly
Atrophic tongue papillae	Iron, vitamin B, vitamin B12, folic acid (but also with antibiotics)
Blue-tinged sclera	Iron

Nutritional Assessment

however, the findings are rarely diagnostic. For example a dry scaly skin is common in sick people who have lost weight; thinning of the skin with easy bruising is seen most often as a result of ageing, and disorders of pigmentation are more often due to systemic disease than to nutritional deficiency.

Atrophy of the tongue papillae together with a variable degree of inflammation may indicate long-standing deficiencies of iron, folic acid or vitamin B complex. Glossitis also occurs commonly after treatment with broad-spectrum antibiotics and may be associated with *Candida* infection.

Aphthous ulcers of the mouth are associated with disorders of the small intestine, especially with Crohn's disease and coeliac disease. They may be associated with marginal deficiencies of iron and folic acid and improve on treatment with these nutrients.

MAJOR STRUCTURAL MINERALS

The human body is usually well supplied with the major structural minerals calcium, magnesium and phosphorus. These minerals are found particularly in the skeleton which to some extent acts as a store for the rest of the body. Deficiency syndromes are difficult to define because they often occur as the result of complex metabolic disorders in sick patients rather than as a response to inadequate intake.

Calcium

The body is capable of adapting to a wide range of intake of calcium (adult intakes vary from less than 400 to over 1600 mg/day). It is suggested that poor adaptation to a prolonged low intake of calcium may be a cause of osteoporosis and that those best able to adapt had a poor intake of calcium in childhood. In the management of the individual patient this statement is not very useful. Hypocalcaemia is not caused by a simple deficiency of calcium. Indeed, hypoproteinaemia is the most common cause as approximately 40% of the circulating mineral is protein bound. Ideally, the clinician needs a measure of ionized calcium which is not readily available from most laboratories. A rough but useful estimation may be obtained from the formula:

Corrected calcium (mmol/l) = Measured calcium (mmol/l) + 0.025 (36 − albumin (g/l))

Ionized calcium is usually held within a narrow range. Low levels occur with vitamin D deficiency, especially in the presence of hypomagnesaemia and in hypoparathyroidism. Calcium excretion in the urine varies widely between normal individuals but is usually low in severe long-standing malabsorption irrespective of vitamin D status.

Bed-bound patients lose calcium from the skeletal mass and in hypercatabolic states the rate of mobilization of calcium from bone may be sufficiently rapid to cause persistent mild hypercalcaemia. This loss of body calcium cannot be prevented by nutritional means.

Phosphorus

Phosphorus is a universal constituent of living cells. It is always present in adequate amounts in a natural diet. Phosphate depletion impairs the metabolism of glucose and may contribute to tissue anoxia by its effect on red cell function. Muscle weakness is a dominant symptom and may cause respiratory failure by its effect on the diaphragm. In prolonged low grade deficiency, the skeleton may become malacic. (This is not surprising because laboratory animals have to be deprived of phosphate as well as of vitamin D in order to produce experimental rickets.)

Low circulating phosphate may occur in subjects taking excessive antacids which precipitate phosphates in the gut, in uncontrolled metabolic acidosis (which causes renal loss of phosphate) and with severe respiratory alkalosis (which is associated with a transcellular phosphate shift, Table 3.10).

In hospital practice, intravenous administration of large quantities of glucose is the most common cause of hypophosphataemia. Insulin transports glucose and phosphate into muscle and liver and this can lead to dangerously low levels of circulating phosphate in periods of rapid refeeding.

Routine tests by the clinical biochemist usually alert the clinician to phosphate depletion before there are serious symptoms. Correction of causative factors (see Table 3.10) is often sufficient treatment, but with very low levels of circulating phosphate (less than 0.5 mmol/l) it may be necessary to supplement intake.

Oral phosphate preparations are not always well tolerated by sick patients. Intravenous infusion may be necessary, especially if circulat-

Nutritional Assessment

Table 3.10 *Causes and treatment of hypophosphataemia*

Effects
  Depletion of cellular ATP (impairing cellular energy) and red cell 2,3-diphosphoglycerate (may cause tissue anoxia)

Causes
  Poor intake/absorption
    Starvation
    Phosphate-binding antacids
    Malabsorption
  Increased losses (renal/non-renal)
    Renal tubular disease (Fanconi's syndrome)
    Acidaemia
    Hyperparathyroidism
    Postrenal transplant
  Transcellular shift (important in clinically significant situations)
    Caused by activation of cellular phosphorylation, e.g. rapid refeeding of a sick phosphate-depleted patient; giving fructose to fructose-intolerant subject. Also occurs in severe alkalosis
  Multifactorial
    Diabetic keto-acidosis
    Chronic alcoholism
    Alcohol withdrawal
    Recovery from burns, trauma, acute pancreatitis

Treatment
  Recognise those at risk
  Correct underlying condition
  Phosphate therapy if serum level very low, e.g. <0.33 mmol/l (1 mg/dl)
  Dose—empirical (stores uncertain), may give a severely hypophosphataemic adult 30–90 mmol over 24 h

---

ing levels are very low and there are signs of damage to the CNS (fits or deteriorating consciousness).

Magnesium

Nearly one-half of the body magnesium is extraskeletal. It is important for the activity of many enzymes and for neuromuscular transmission. The circulating concentration (of which 55% is ionic) is not under hormonal control and thus provides a reasonable index of body status. Magnesium deficiency is not uncommon in hospital practice. It occurs especially with serious small intestinal disease (Crohn's disease, coeliac disease and small intestinal resection), and as a result of renal tubular dysfunction which may be caused by alcohol, by some drugs (aminoglycosides, Amphotericin B and possibly cytotoxic agents) and by the prolonged use of diuretics. The symptoms may include anorexia, nausea, tremors, tetany (with associated hypocalcaemia and often hypokalaemic alkalosis) and cardiac dysrhythmias. It is important to monitor circulating calcium, magnesium and phosphate in patients with prolonged illnesses particularly if there is associated gastrointestinal, hepatic or renal dysfunction or if management involves the use of cytoxic agents and antibiotics for recurrent infections (Table 3.11).

A serum magnesium level of less than 0.5 mmol/l or a urine excretion of less than 0.5 mmol/24 h usually indicates serious depletion. In doubtful cases the response to treatment may be helpful in determining the significance of borderline laboratory results. It is important, however, to remember that hypomagnesaemia rarely if ever causes recognizable symptoms unless the body is deficient of other nutrients, especially calcium and potassium.

EXTRACELLULAR SUPPORTING TISSUE – THE FLUID COMPARTMENT

In undertaking a nutritional assessment one must consider body fluids, the volume and composition of which often undergo major changes during acute illness. Detailed analysis of water and electrolyte balance are outside the scope of this book. Common problems occurring with malnutrition are discussed briefly below. For a more comprehensive coverage of the problems of body salt and water the reader should consult an appropriate monograph (see Further Reading).

Dehydration

In clinical practice the term dehydration is used to describe the pathophysiological changes produced by a reduction in the volume of extracellular fluid (ECF). A dehydrated patient is usually short of both salt and water; a reduction of body water alone is uncommon.

Saline deficiency

Loss of salt and water reduces the volume of plasma and ECF. With early depletion, symptoms are non-specific. The patient complains of

Table 3.11 *Causes and treatment of hypomagnesaemia*

Effects
  Magnesium depletion inhibits many enzyme systems, especially those using ATP. This may affect membrane permeability, neuromuscular excitability, synthesis of protein fat and nucleic acids, and oxidative phosphorylation

Causes
  Poor intake/absorption
    Dietary Kwashiorkor*
    Malabsorption*
  Increased renal losses
    Renal disease
      Renal tubular acidosis
      Diuretic phase of acute tubular necrosis
    Drugs
      Diuretics
      Aminoglycosides
      Cytotoxic agents
      Amphotericin B*
  Increased gastrointestinal losses
    Colitis
    Laxative-induced diarrhoea
    Fistulae
    Short bowel syndrome*

Endocrine and metabolic disorders
    Hyperparathyroidism
    Hyperthyroidism
    Hyperaldosteronism
    Diabetic ketoacidosis
    Pancreatitis
    Alcoholism*

Management
  Recognise those at risk
  Correct underlying condition
  Mild deficiency—high Mg diet (meat, dairy products, cereals, green vegetables)
  Moderate deficiency—oral supplements of salts most easily absorbed, e.g. Mg gluconate
  Severe deficiency—i.v. Mg 20–40 mmol over 12 h

Note
  Often have to treat associated deficiencies, e.g. potassium

*Indicates clinically common causes.

being tired and weak; later he may be thirsty. The clinician must look for significant signs in those at risk. The fall in ECF volume causes:

Sudden weight loss (hence the value of weighing sick patients daily)
Low central venous pressure
Postural hypotension (sign of uncertain value in the elderly)
Oliguria (the urine is usually but not necessarily highly concentrated)

In clinical practice the conventional signs of dehydration are rarely useful. They include a reduction in tissue turgor which is difficult to distinguish from the effects of wasting (especially in older patients), a dry mouth which is usually caused by mouth breathing or a failure of salivation and not by dehydration, and reduced intraocular pressure (only recognizable in the very depleted). On the other hand, in infants a sunken anterior fontanelle may be a valuable physical sign of salt and water depletion.

Laboratory measurements are of most value when obtained sequentially. The haematocrit falls (with a rise in haemoglobin concentration), the blood urea may rise (but the actual concentration depends on renal function and protein intake) and the concentration of sodium in urine falls to less than 20 mmol/l.

Water deficiency

A deficit of water is distributed over both intra- and extracellular fluid and thus ECF volume is reasonably well maintained. The patient is thirsty and may become confused. In contrast to the effects of saline deficiency, the plasma osmolality increases and hypernatraemia develops. The urine is also highly concentrated (more than 700 mmol/kg).

Overhydration

Overhydration most commonly occurs against a background of chronic pathology, such as congestive cardiac failure, cirrhosis and conditions causing hypoalbuminaemia (such as nephrosis). In these situations both salt and water are retained.

Simple excess of water may occur with the infusion of too much hypotonic fluid too quickly, with compulsive water drinking, during a drinking binge with an excessive intake of a weak solution of alcohol (e.g. beer), or as a result of the injudicious use of water enemas (especially in a patient with an enlarged colon). Water intoxication may also occur as a result of the ineffective clearance of water by the kidneys. This may result from an 'inappropriate' secretion of antidiuretic hormone (ADH). It occurs in some acute illnesses (especially intracerebral and pulmonary), as a result of ectopic secretion of ADH by neoplastic tissue and with deficiency of thyroid or adrenocorticoid hormones.

Saline excess

An excess of saline leads to an increased body weight, a high central venous pressure (unless the plasma albumin is low) and oedema (which appears when fluid and salt retention exceeds 5–10% of normal body weight). The patient may develop effusions in serous cavities, pulmonary congestion and signs of cardiac failure.

Water excess

The water-intoxicated patient develops cerebral oedema. This may cause confusion and, in the later stages, impaired consciousness. In the early phase of water-intoxication, weight is increased, serum sodium is reduced and urine is very dilute provided that the secretion of ADH has been suppressed. Paradoxically, the expanded ECF maintains the excretion of sodium despite the hyponatraemia.

BODY CHLORIDE

Because it is no longer measured routinely, chloride is rarely considered in nutritional assessment. Body chloride is predominantly an extracellular ion with a plasma concentration of 100–106 mmol/l. It is present in low concentrations in bone and connective tissue where it is loosely bound and readily exchangeable. Deficiency usually occurs in association with sodium although recurrent vomiting will cause a differential loss of chloride ions. This is important as the concomitant potassium deficiency cannot be corrected without an infusion of adequate amounts of chloride. Hyperchloraemia is rarely an isolated problem but may occur with excess chloride absorption from the colon in the patient with a uretero-intestinal anastomosis.

VITAMINS AND TRACE ELEMENTS

In hospital practice, detailed assessment of the nutritional state of the body with respect to vitamins and trace elements apart from iron is not usually undertaken. Severe deficiencies causing overt signs occur rarely. Minor deficiencies may be recognized biochemically but the results of special tests are often difficult to interpret and often are of doubtful clinical significance. The methods available are summarized in Tables 3.12 and 3.13.

PUTTING THEORY INTO PRACTICE

The signs and symptoms of severe malnutrition are not difficult to recognize (Table 3.14). On the other hand, lesser degrees of nutritional dysfunction may be difficult to disentangle from the effects of primary pathology. In such cases the clinician often decides to provide supplementary nutritional support without good evidence that this will improve prognosis.

When a case of nutritional difficiency is suspected, it is important to follow a logical sequence of steps:

1. Take a clinical history to elucidate disorders likely to be associated with nutritional deficiency, e.g.:
   (a) Psychosocial factors (see Table 5.1, p. 134)
   (b) Loss of appetite
   (c) Gastrointestinal disease, especially if associated with nausea, vomiting, diarrhoea or jaundice
   (d) Blood loss
   (e) Metabolic disorders
   (f) Infective, inflammatory or neoplastic pathology, especially when this is associated with weight loss
2. Take a dietary history to identify:
   (a) Anorexia as a cause of weight loss (especially if this is 10% or more of normal weight)
   (b) Specific deficiencies
3. A clinical examination should be performed to assess:
   (a) Body weight (compare with normal weight and ideal weight)
   (b) Fat stores and skeletal muscle mass (measure muscle strength but be aware of non-nutritional factors)

Table 3.12 Vitamin deficiencies—diagnosis and significance

Vitamin	Deficiency disease	Laboratory assessment	Significance
Vitamin A	Night blindness Xerophthalmia	Plasma retinol Retinol binding protein	Low-grade deficiency in malabsorptive disorders Major problem in the Third World
Vitamin B			
Thiamin (B1)	Peripheral neuropathy Cardiac failure Wernicke–Korsakoff syndrome (especially in alcoholics)	Red cell transketolase Glucose challenge (lactate, pyruvate accumulate)	Problem in poorly-nourished alcoholics
Riboflavin (B2)	Isolated deficiency only in experiments (seborrhoea, glossitis, anaemia)	Red cell glutathione reductase	Only as part of generalised vitamin B deficiency
Niacin (B3)	Pellagra Light-sensitive rash Watery diarrhoea Disturbed cerebration	Urinary methyl nicotinamide	Rare in developed countries (occasionally in carcinoid syndrome and with isoniazid therapy)
Pyridoxine (B6)	Sideroblastic anaemia	Circulating pyridoxal phosphate	Very rare, ? significance of low levels with pill
Biotin (B8)	Very rare skin disorder in infants (Leiner's disease)	Circulating levels	Not described (except in unsupplemented total parenteral nutrition (TPN))
Vitamin C (ascorbate)	Scurvy	Leucocyte concentrations	Rare except food faddism
Vitamin D	Rickets/osteomalacia Myopathy	25 HO-Cholecalciferol	Low-grade deficiency common especially with avoidance sunlight, high fibre diets, anticonvulsants
Vitamin E	Infants only Spinocerebellar disorders Haemolysis	Plasma a-Tocopherol Ability of red cells to withstand oxidant stress	Only with severe fat malabsorption—obstructive jaundice from birth
Vitamin K	Bleeding diathesis	Prothrombin time	Clinical deficiency with steatorrhoea and obstructive jaundice

Table 3.13 Trace element deficiencies—diagnosis and significance

Trace element	Deficiency disease	Laboratory investigation	Significance
Zinc	Peristomal and acral dermatitis (bullous/pustular eruption)	Plasma zinc (uncertain value)	Rare congenital disorder Occasionally in TPN
	? Failure of growth		In Middle East
Copper	Anaemia Hair changes in infants	Plasma copper in relation to caeruloplasmin	Rare congenital disorder Occasionally in TPN
Chromium	Glucose intolerance Neuropathy	Plasma and hair values (only patchy data)	Possible with long-standing TPN
Selenium	? Cardiomyopathy (Keshan's disease)	Plasma glutathione oxidase	Uncertain
Vanadium	Uncertain ?oedema	Methods unreliable	Nil at present
Molybdenum	Encephalopathy	High urinary xanthine, hypoxanthine	Long-standing TPN (one case)
Iodine	Goitre Thyroid insufficiency	Thyroid function	Influenced by dietary and environmental factors

    (c) Signs of possible protein, trace element and vitamin deficiencies (see Tables 3.12, 3.13). The clinical findings are often non-specific but may serve to remind the clinician of the need to ensure an adequate supply of nutrients during periods of prolonged ill-health
    (d) Body fluids (see point 4(b) overleaf)
4. Laboratory tests should be carried out to provide a measure of:
    (a) Haematological variables and haematinic status

Table 3.14 Nutritional assessment—summary of methods

Factors	Routine assessment	Readily available tests	Special investigations
Body build	Clinical impression; height weight (compare ideal and previous)	Waist: hip ratio—measure of distribution of body fat	
Body composition			
Fat	Clinical assessment	Skinfold thickness	Isotope methods
Protein		Simple nitrogen balance	Body water, nitrogen, potassium
Active tissue mass			
Skeletal muscle	Clinical assessment	Muscle circumference, area Grip strength	Muscle stimulation tests Histology
Liver	Clinical (e.g. jaundice, oedema) LFTs, PT, circulating proteins	Clearance and breath tests	Tests of intermediary metabolism
Blood	Full blood count Examination of blood film	Iron/IBC Folate/RBC folate, B12	Ferritin Marrow morphology
Immune system	Lymphocyte count Circulating immunoglobulins	(Delayed hypersensitivity skin tests)	Secretory IgG T and B cells
Heart	Clinical assessment	ECG	
CNS	Clinical assessment	EMG, EEG	
Supporting tissues			
Hair, skin, nails, mucous membranes	Clinical assessment		Tests of protein, vitamin, trace element, EFA status
Skeleton	Clinical assessment Circulating Ca, P, Alk. phos.	Further radiology	Bone biopsy, 25–HOCC
Plasma	Clinical assessment Circulating urea/electrolytes	Direct measurements CVP	Isotope methods
Specific factors			
Vitamins	Clinical assessment Effects on circulating substances, e.g. Ca, P, AP (vitamin D); Prothrombin (vitamin K)	Response to treatment	Red cell enzymes (vitamin B) Leucocyte vitamin C Retinol/RBP (vitamin A)
Minerals	Radiology skeleton Plasma Ca, Mg, P	Tests of neuromuscular excitability	Isotope methods
Trace elements	Clinical assessment	Serum zinc	Other trace elements

(b) Fluid and electrolyte balance (clinical assessment in the light of laboratory measurement)
(c) Status with respect to divalent cations (iron, calcium, magnesium, zinc) and circulating phosphate
(d) Circulating proteins and enzymes (e.g. alkaline phosphatase) The values obtained can be assessed only with a full knowledge of associated pathology
(e) Circulating lipids

5. Radiological, scanning and isotope studies, and tissue biopsies are rarely needed. They are occasionally helpful in the assessment of:
(a) Nutritional bone disorders
(b) Effects of malnutrition on organ structure (e.g. muscle, liver)
(c) Research investigations

In order to confirm a suspected case of nutritional deficiency, it may be necessary to undertake special tests (see Table 3.14) or to treat the patient and observe the results. Sequential observations are of considerable value (see Table 5.8, p. 151). Clinicians must also be aware of unusual disorders (e.g. deficiencies of trace elements or of essential fatty acids which may develop in patients with prolonged illness).

FURTHER READING

Baker J. P., Detsky A. S., Weeson D. E., et al. (1982). Nutritional assessment: a comparison of clinical judgement and objective measurements. *New Engl. J. Med*; **306**: 969–72.

Bamji M. S. (1981). Laboratory tests for the assessment of vitamin nutritional status. In *Vitamins in Human Biology and Medicine*. (Briggs M. H., ed.) Boca Taton, Florida: CRC Press Inc.

Heymsfield S. B., McManus C., Smith J., Stevens V., Nixon D. W. (1982). Anthropometric measurement of muscle mass: revised equations for calculating bone-free arm muscle area. *Amer. J. Clin. Nut*; **38**: 680–90.

Keys A., Brozek K., Henschel A., Mickelson O., Taylor H. L. (1950). *The Biology of Human Starvation*. Minneapolis: University of Minnesota Press.

Neale G., Elia M. (1986). Nutritional assessment. In *Clinical Nutrition in Gastroenterology*, Chapter 4, pp. 82–98. (Heatley V., Kelleher J., Losowsky M., eds.) Edinburgh: Churchill Livingstone.

Richards P., Truniger B. (1983). *Understanding Water, Electrolyte and Acid–Base Balance*. London: William Heinemann Medical Books.

Solomons N. W., Allan L. H. (1983). The functional assessment of nutritional status: principles, practice and potential. *Nut. Rev*; **41**: 33–50.

Chapter 4

Recognition and Management of Nutritional Disorders

DEFICIENCY DISORDERS ● ANOREXIA NERVOSA ● NUTRITIONAL ANAEMIAS ● NUTRITIONAL DEFICIENCIES AFFECTING THE SKELETON ● NUTRITIONAL DEFICIENCIES IN ALCOHOLICS ● MALNUTRITION IN SUBJECTS TAKING SPECIFIC DIETS ● DRUGS PREDISPOSING TO NUTRIENT DEFICIENCIES ● OBESITY ● HYPERLIPIDAEMIA ● DIET IN THE MANAGEMENT OF SPECIFIC DISEASE ● FURTHER READING

Diet is an important form of treatment. It may be vital to the patient's health, as in coeliac disease; it may complement other forms of treatment, as in renal or hepatic failure, and it is nearly always a matter of concern to patients ('What shall I eat doctor?').

In this chapter we shall consider the principles of management of a variety of conditions in which diet has an important role.

DEFICIENCY DISORDERS

Protein-energy malnutrition (PEM)

Throughout the world as a whole, PEM is undoubtedly the most common nutritional disorder. As the name implies the disease is due to an inadequate intake of protein and energy. The classical disorders, marasmus and Kwashiorkor, were defined in studies of infants in the developing countries. More recently a similar technology has been used to describe adults who have lost weight as a result of serious pathology. In consequence, there have been many reports claiming to show protein-energy malnutrition in 25–50% of medical and surgical patients who have illnesses requiring admission to hospital for 2 weeks or more. By implication it is suggested that the prevention or treatment of this 'malnutrition' will improve prognosis. Such statements must be interpreted with care. Loss of weight in the patient with chronic disease may be an adaptive response. It should not be equated directly with the effects of semistarvation. Or again, hypoalbuminaemia is rarely due to nutritional deficiency alone (see Chapter 3, p. 60). Thus it is frankly misleading to use the term Kwashiorkor without careful analysis of possible causes of hypoproteinaemia. Confusion is avoided by careful use of terminology and by describing pathological processes rather than using diagnostic labels.

Marasmus

Clinicians interested in the disorders of childhood have used the term marasmus for more than a century. It has its roots in the Greek word *marasmos* – a dying away. It has been applied to severe malnutrition occurring especially in the first year of life. It is characterized by growth retardation and progressive wasting. The child has a good or even voracious appetite and remains remarkably alert. The starving children of central Africa show the classical signs of marasmus (Fig. 4.1a).

Kwashiorkor (Fig. 4.1b)

In 1931 Cicely Williams introduced the word Kwashiorkor into modern medicine (Annual Medical Report of The Gold Coast Colony). The original description of the disorder is quoted (Williams, 1933) in order to try to improve clinical understanding.

> 'It (Kwashiorkor) occurs in children between the ages of 1 and 4 years in whom there is a history of deficient breast feeding. The only supplementary food used is a preparation of maize. The disease takes from 4 to 12 months to declare itself.
>
> The lesions of the skin are extensive, well-marked and characteristic. They may be accompanied by oedema of the extremities. The mucous membranes are often inflamed and ulcerated. There is a tendency to vomiting and in chronic cases wasting may be severe. Diarrhoea occurs and may become persistent. The stools show undigested food but no ova or parasites. The child is extremely irritable and may die in a few days if not treated. It has been impossible to conduct a scientific investigation into the cause or to

Recognition and Management of Nutritional Disorders 85

make controlled experiments into the nature of the cure. But the similarity of this condition with other deficiency diseases suggests that the remedy should be dietetic. My general impression is that cod liver oil and a good brand of tinned milk are the most important elements of treatment. Cod liver oil seems to delay the onset of the fulminating phase; but only with inpatients, for whom an adequate supply of good milk can be assured, is a cure established. At post-mortem nothing characteristic is found except a very fatty almost diffluent liver. Several aetiological factors may play a part in this syndrome. As maize is the only source of supplementary food, some amino acid or protein deficiency cannot be excluded as a cause. . . .

Maize is deficient in tryptophan, lysine and glycine.'

Cicely Williams took the term Kwashiorkor from the language of the Ga tribe who live around Accra. They used the name for 'the sickness the older child gets when the next baby is born'. Williams had no doubt that she was treating a nutritional disorder associated with inappropriate feeding after weaning and indeed her classical article is headed *Nutritional (Maize) Disease.*

It is extraordinary that these beautiful observations were ignored for 20 years. In Africa the disease became confused with pellagra until 1952 when the FAO/WHO Expert Committee on Nutrition commissioned an enquiry into the features of Kwashiorkor. The term protein-calorie malnutrition was then introduced because severely malnourished children could not be characterized simply. The range of clinical appearance was too wide. Many workers emphasized oedema, depigmentation and hair changes as part of the Kwashiorkor syndrome. Cicely Williams did not. To quote again:

'Any African child who suffers from chronic disease generally shows some degree of depigmentation. The child who in health would be rich black or dark glossy brown gradually becomes a dull reddish muddy colour. The hair in a disease such as profound helminthiasis becomes dry pale and sparse. . . .'

Again '. . . there may be oedema . . .'. One suspects that the infants she describes were all hypoalbuminaemic, but even in malnourished children this is not the sole determining factor for oedema.

The understanding of protein malnutrition was not helped by the report of an international working party sponsored by the Wellcome Trust. This group formulated a classification of malnutrition based solely on the presence or absence of oedema and deficit of body weight. A *Lancet* editorial commented that widespread acceptance of this simple classification would greatly ease the comparison of and investigation of malnutrition in various parts of the world. It is still widely used even though the classification ignores clinical reality. A child with dietary Kwashiorkor who is not too ill responds readily to dietary supplements containing first class protein. Such a response will not be seen in the underweight child who develops oedema as a result of a defined pathology, such as measles, hookworm infection or the nephrotic syndrome. It would help if the terms maramus and Kwashiorkor were limited solely to the effects of severe nutritional deficiency.

The nature of marasmus and Kwashiorkor has been explored in experimental animals. Marasmus (generalized wasting) occurs with simple reduction of food intake. In growing animals, this leads to a failure of growth and developmental retardation (Fig. 4.2b). In contrast, Kwashiorkor is produced by allowing animals unlimited intake of a diet with a low protein-energy ratio particularly when the protein is poor in one or more essential amino acids. Excess energy elevates blood glucose which leads to hyperinsulinaemia and the deposition of fat. It promotes the synthesis of muscle protein which in turn increases the requirement for essential amino acids. If these are in short supply, muscle competes with other organs especially the liver. The hepatic synthesis of export proteins, such as albumin and the lipoproteins is reduced in an animal eating a diet with a low protein-energy ratio. Thus, like the child with Kwashiorkor, the experimental animal becomes hypoalbuminaemic and develops a fatty liver.

There is considerable species to species variation in the ability of animals to adapt to low protein-high energy diets. Rats are particularly poor models and have to be fed a diet virtually free of protein before developing a Kwashiorkor-like picture. Man too may vary in his response. Dietary Kwashiorkor is seen only in parts of the world where the main source of protein is particularly poor in quality, e.g. the maize pap described by Cicely Williams in Ghana and the cassava and plantain diet of large areas in central Africa where the energy intake is adequate or even high.

A Kwashiorkor-like syndrome occurs rarely in the Western World. It has been described in patients with severe malabsorption of protein who are nevertheless obtaining sufficient calories. This may occur in the gastrectomized patient who develops pancreatic insufficiency. Protein cannot be absorbed without digestion by pepsin or trypsin but

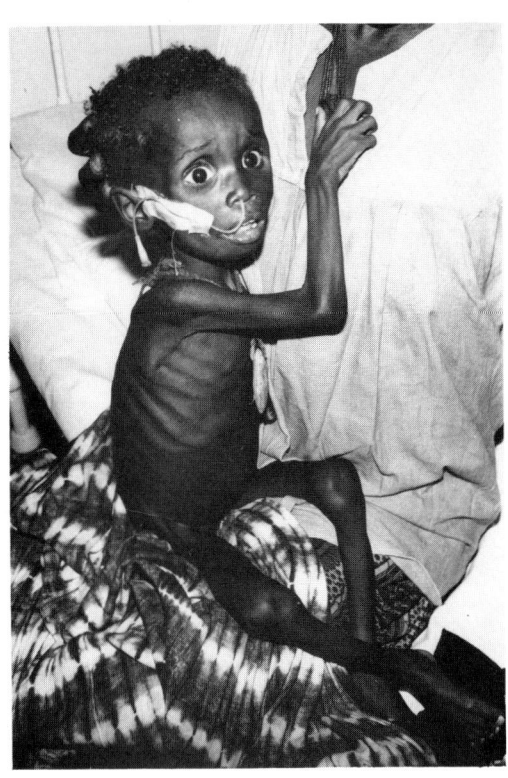

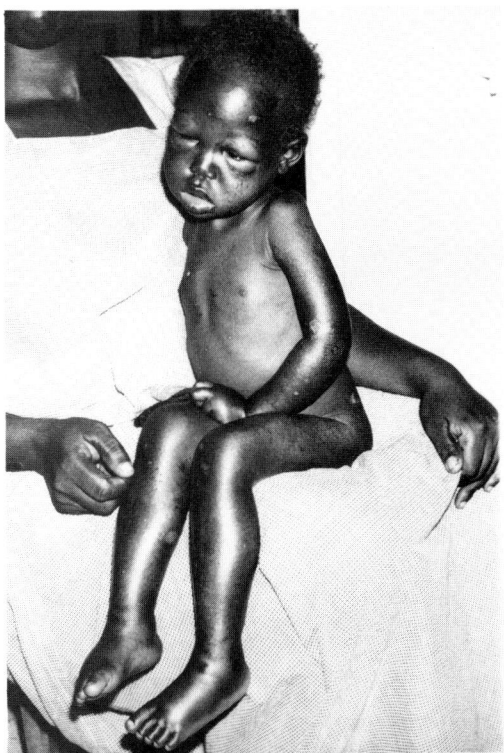

Figure 4.1a and b. The dramatic clinical difference between marasmus (Fig. 4.1a) and Kwashiorkor (Fig. 4.16). (Photographs by kind permission of Dr R. G. Whitehead, Dunn Nutrition|Unit, Addenbrooke's Hospital, Cambridge.)

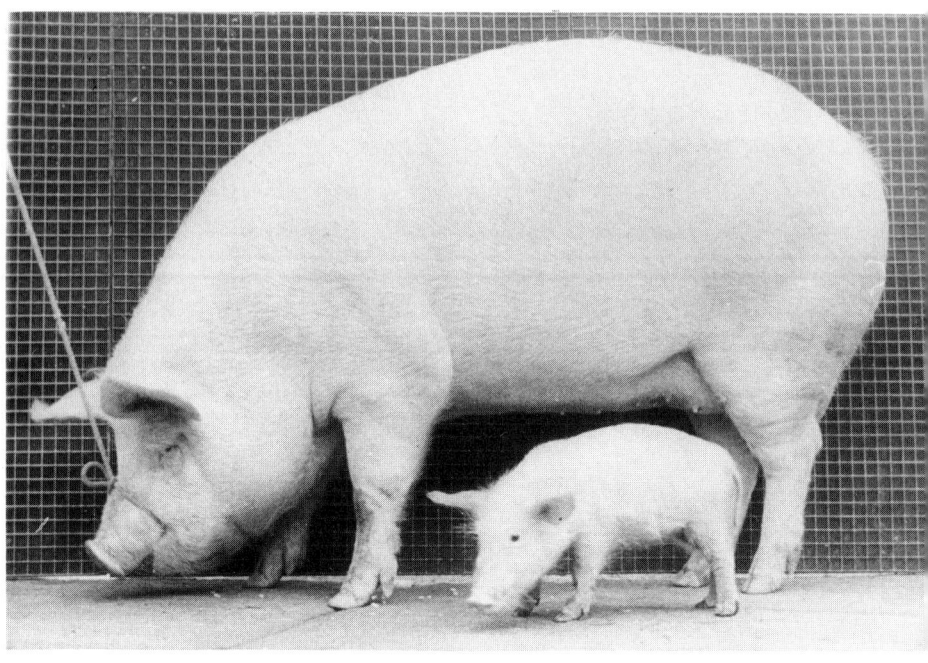

Figure 4.2. The effect of severe undernutrition on growth and development in the experimental animal. The undernourished animal has been given very small amounts of the same diet fed *ad libitum* to its litter mate for 1 year. Its weight is only 3% of normal, the body proportions are incorrect and the animal is sexually immature. Refeeding allows catch-up growth which is less effective the longer the period of malnutrition. Photograph by kind permission of Dr Elsie Widdowson. (From: E. Widdowson. (1964). In *Diet and Bodily Constitution.* Ciba Foundation Study Group. No. 17.)

there will be substantial uptake of carbohydrate (especially disaccharides which are digested by intestinal brush border enzymes). A similar picture may occur in the stagnant loop syndrome because of the metabolism of dietary protein by bacteria. Kwashiorkor-like malnutrition has also been described in artificially fed patients given excessive calories but little protein. Such patients become hypoproteinaemic with fatty livers and develop the irritable apathy described in children with Kwashiorkor. The clinical and biochemical abnormalities respond rapidly to replenishment of the patient with protein.

ANOREXIA NERVOSA

From time to time the clinician with an interest in nutritional disorders will be asked to see a patient (usually an adolescent female) who has anorexia nervosa. This occurs because the parents are striving desperately to ignore the evidence before their eyes and are hoping to be told that their child has a simple organic disorder.

Minor appetite disorders are common at puberty. Girls in our society are under enormous social pressure to be successful (often in an academic sense) at a time when they are developing into womanhood. To compound the problem, obesity is socially unacceptable in adolescence; yet physiologically this is at a time of rapid weight gain.

Often dieting to reduce weight is the trigger factor for anorexia nervosa. Any form of dieting at this age should be carefully supervised. It is all too easy for the young girl to eat less than she needs. She will choose her food for what she perceives as its fattening or slimming properties. She will pay no attention to nutrient content. In most cases the range of food ingested becomes extremely limited. As a result the subject not only loses weight but may also develop deficiencies of minerals and vitamins.

In a minor way the condition may affect as many as 5–10% of schoolgirls between the ages of 16 and 18 years. About one-tenth of these will go on to develop established anorexia nervosa with a morbid fear of overeating, denial of weight loss, devious behaviour and resistance to any form of treatment. Males are much less commonly affected. Some patients resort to bouts of overeating with self-induced vomiting (bulimia) and others to periodic episodes of purgation.

The metabolic and endocrine consequences are different from those of semistarvation perhaps in part because of the curious quality of the diet. Secondary amenorrhoea is almost universal. The breasts and external genitalia atrophy and the skin grows a fine downy hair. Hormone tests show depressed gonadal and thyroid function. Yet glucose tolerance is impaired and circulating cholesterol may rise to high levels. There is often evidence of sodium and potassium depletion but during an episode of refeeding, oedema may appear.

The general physician should have little difficulty in making the correct diagnosis, although the surreptitious use of laxatives and diuretics may produce a misleading picture. If he has the time and patience the general physician should be able to manage a mildly affected patient. Severe and well-established cases are best managed by psychiatrists with a special interest in the condition.

Usually the patient's environment needs to be tightly controlled and the patient's family involved in the treatment. Prolonged admission to a metabolic ward may be necessary for controlled refeeding. In these circumstances, many clinicians use a combination of family psychotherapy and a reward system to reinforce behaviour which encourages an increase in food intake. In some cases life can be maintained only by artificial nutritional support. After discharge from hospital careful follow-up is necessary. Relapse is common and 10–20% of patients will die with their disorder (most often by suicide). The prognosis is particularly poor for the older patient.

NUTRITIONAL ANAEMIAS

Anaemia is a very common nutritional disorder. For effective haematopoiesis the marrow requires adequate supplies of protein, iron, folic acid, vitamin B12, pyridoxine, vitamin C and trace elements.

Iron

For the production of red cells the most common limiting nutritional factor is a deficiency of iron. This is not surprising as the amount of iron which can be absorbed from a normal diet is not much above normal requirements (Fig. 4.3). Iron is best absorbed from the haem of meat (20%), less well from cereals (5–10%) and least well from green vegetables (1–5%). Up to about 4 mg iron a day may be absorbed from the diet; usually it is considerably less.

The patient with an iron deficient anaemia is usually asymptomatic

Recognition and Management of Nutritional Disorders

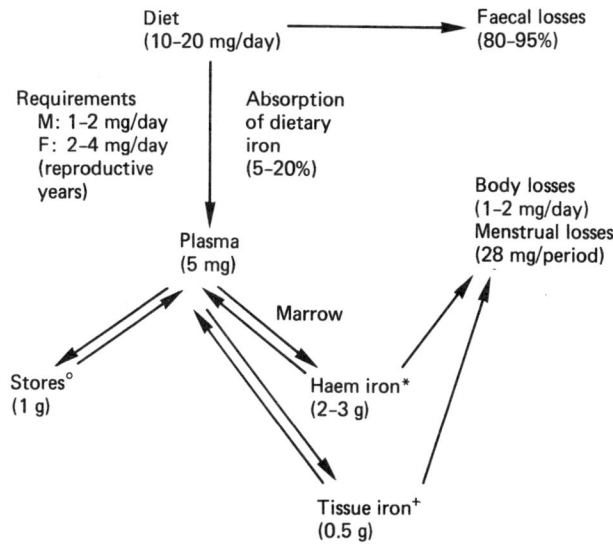

* As haemoglobin
+ As myoglobin, haem enzymes, non-haem enzymes
o In liver, spleen and marrow as ferritin and haemosiderin

Figure 4.3 Iron. Body stores—absorption and excretion.

although after effective treatment there is often a sense of rejuvenation. Iron deficiency may be caused by:

1. Poor dietary intake.
2. Malabsorption, e.g. post-gastrectomy, coeliac disease.
3. Increased demands, e.g. of chronic blood loss due to: heavy menstruation, gastrointestinal pathology, the taking of NSAID; also the increased demands of repeated pregnancy.

In assessing the iron-deficient patient all these factors should be considered. It is necessary to look carefully for hidden pathology. Delay in diagnosis occurs most frequently with cancer of the caecum and coeliac disease. Iron deficiency in a previously fit man over the age of 50 is most often due to occult blood loss from the intestine (especially the colon). In women of similar age, it may be due to long-standing depletion because of a negative iron balance during the reproductive years. It is difficult to replete the body with iron by simple dietary means because the absorption of organic iron is relatively poor. Thus women may be unable to catch up on their physiological losses.

In young people recurrent iron deficiency may be the only sign of coeliac disease. A biopsy of jejunal mucosa is indicated if the dietary intake is adequate and if there is no evidence of excess blood loss from the intestine. In some cases, the cause of iron deficiency remains uncertain even after detailed investigation. For example, it is particularly difficult to identify recurrent small bleeds from an angiodysplastic lesion in the intestine. It may be necessary to replete iron stores and then to see the patient at intervals (3–6 months) to determine whether or not deficiency is going to recur. After such treatment a small percentage of patients remain well and the cause of their iron deficiency remains undetermined. The iron deficient patient requires treatment with an appropriate inorganic salt (ferrous sulphate is cheap and effective). The medication should be taken daily for 3 months in order to replete iron stores. Treatment for too short a time is a common cause of recurrent low grade iron deficiency anaemia. After partial gastrectomy or intestinal resection a liquid iron preparation is more effective than tablets because these can pass through to the colon unchanged. If the anaemia fails to respond to treatment it is important to check that there is no associated cause (such as hidden inflammatory disease suppressing haematopoiesis) and that iron stores have been repleted. To continue to give iron indefinitely to an anaemic patient is not only poor medical practice but may culminate in a potentially dangerous iron overload.

Folic acid

Folate occurs in most natural foodstuffs in a variety of forms of conjugated pteroyl-polyglutamate. A normal diet contains about 300 μg total folate/day of which a proportion has to be broken down to the monoglutamate before absorption. (The enzyme, folate conjugase, is found in the intestinal mucosa and in some foods.)

The folate compounds differ in their chemical stability and biological potency. They are needed for the transfer of one-carbon units as formyl ($-CHO$) or methyl ($-CH_3$) groups. This process is particularly important for the synthesis of the purines and pyrimidines of nucleic acid.

A normal adult has sufficient stores of folate to meet requirements for 2–3 months. Depletion leads to a megaloblastic anaemia which affects the synthesis of all marrow components. Glossitis and mucosal changes in the intestine also occur because of the high rate of turnover of gut mucosal cells. Folate deficiency occurs as a result of:

1. Nutritional deficiency – especially in the elderly, in pregnant women and low birth weight infants.
2. Malabsorption – especially in coeliac disease.
3. Interference with metabolism – e.g. by alcohol, or anticonvulsants.
4. Increased requirements – whenever there is rapid cell growth or turnover, e.g. in pregnancy, in haemolytic disorders and in patients with exfoliative dermatitis.

Measurement of red cell folate is the most sensitive method of assessing folic acid status. Before treatment with folic acid it is important to ensure that the patient is not vitamin B12 deficient. Long-term treatment of the B12 deficient patient with folic acid will correct the megaloblastic anaemia but will not prevent subacute combined degeneration of the spinal cord.

Folic acid deficiency is readily treated. A dose of 5 mg folic acid one to three times a day is sufficient to meet requirements in all situations.

Vitamin B12

Vitamin B12 (cobalamin) is produced by bacteria. Man obtains his B12 preformed in foods of animal origin. He requires no more than 1–2 µg/day and most B12 in food is available for absorption. A good quality mixed diet may contain as much as 50 µg/day. A strict vegetarian (vegan) diet contains virtually no vitamin B12 (only minimal amounts come from bacterial contamination) and will lead ultimately to B12 deficiency.

Dietary vitamin B12 is released in the stomach to become bound to a secreted glycoprotein called intrinsic factor (IF). The B12–IF complex passes to the ileum where it attaches to specific receptors for absorption. In the normal adult, sufficient B12 is stored in the liver to provide for up to 3–5 years. Vitamin B12 acts with folic acid in the synthesis of nucleic acid. Depletion of the vitamin leads to a megaloblastic anaemia indistinguishable from that caused by folate deficiency. In addition, B12 is required for the integrity of the nervous system. Peripheral neuropathy and subacute combined degeneration of the spinal cord occur with prolonged deficiency. Deficiency of vitamin B12 is caused by:

1. A vegan diet.
2. Failure of secretion of IF (pernicious anaemia, gastric resection).
3. Bacterial uptake of vitamin B12 (in the stagnant loop syndrome).
4. Ileal disorders (e.g. after intestinal resection, and rarely with ileal Crohn's disease).

Intramuscular hydroxycobalamin 1000 µg every 3 months provides adequate treatment.

Other haematinics

Pyridoxine (vitamin B6) is essential for the synthesis of haem by acting as a coenzyme for D-amino-laevulinate synthetase. Dietary deficiency is virtually unknown. Reduced values of circulating pyridoxal phosphate have been described in severe malabsorption and in alcoholics.

The hypochromic anaemia of unknown aetiology which occurs in association with a sideroblastic bone marrow sometimes responds to treatment with pyridoxine. In such cases, the enzyme D-amino-laevulinate synthetase appears to have a markedly reduced affinity for its coenzyme. Treatment with large doses of pyridoxine (500 mg/day) is sometimes effective.

Ascorbic acid (vitamin C) deficiency is usually associated with anaemia. It occurs with long-standing poor dietary intake. In nearly all cases there is an associated folate deficiency. The anaemia is multifactorial – bleeding, haemolysis and depression of marrow function all play a part. Patients respond rapidly to treatment with ascorbic acid and folate.

The role of trace elements in haematopoiesis in man is uncertain. Copper may be needed for the adequate absorption or utilization of iron. Deficiency has been described in rural communities in some developing countries. It could also occur in patients on long-standing parenteral nutrition because requirements in sick people are uncertain.

NUTRITIONAL DEFICIENCIES AFFECTING THE SKELETON

Osteopenia is a clinical disorder of great and increasing concern with huge economic consequences. Health and social services devote an increasing proportion of their resources to the care of the frail elderly. It is estimated that one in three women will suffer the effects of post menopausal osteoporosis: one in five will fracture their hips or vertebrae.

Loss of bone with increasing age is universal but it begins earlier and develops more rapidly in women than in men. Most patients with osteoporosis present with bone pain or fracture, by which time bone loss is considerable and largely irreversible. Osteopenia is not primarily a nutritional disorder (Table 4.1), although vitamin D status and

Table 4.1 *Factors affecting bone mass*

1. Peak bone mass at maturity
    Genetic factors
    Environmental factors
        Exercise
        Dietary calcium
        Vitamin D status
2. Age-related bone atrophy
    Genetic factors
    Endocrine factors acting on
        Bone modelling
            Perimenopausal osteoporosis
            (? role of oestrogens)
        Calcium absorption
            ? low 1:25 di–HOCC
            ? end organ senescence
            ? increased PTH
    Environmental factors
        Decreased mobility
        Reduced calcium intake

calcium intake are significant modulating factors. The size and structure of the skeleton result largely from an interaction between genetic make-up, mechanical demands and hormonal influences. In some circumstances, the availability of calcium and vitamin D act as limiting factors. Other factors which may affect bone mass adversely include caffeine (calciuric effect), smoking and a heavy intake of alcohol. Conversely, fluoride in drinking water (1 mg/l) tends to be protective and the obese have stronger bones than the lean.

Firm guidelines for the improvement of skeletal mass are lacking.

Hormonal replacement (e.g. ethinyl oestriol 25 mg daily for 3 weeks in every 4) is undoubtedly valuable in the management of perimenopausal osteoporosis and should be used in all women with premature ovarian failure. But this is only a small percentage of those at risk. At present there is no good method of identifying women who will develop osteoporosis after a natural menopause.

Treatment is usually delayed until presentation with fractures after minimal trauma. Most authorities advise treatment with oestrogen for 5–10 years. Such treatment may also offer some protection against atheroma. Whether or not it increases the risk of endometrial or breast carcinoma is uncertain. For osteoporosis of the elderly, treatment is even less certain. Nevertheless, in both groups it is sensible to check on dietary intakes of calcium and the patient's vitamin D status. It has been suggested that recommended levels of calcium intake should be boosted to 25 mmol (1100 mg) for women approaching the menopause and to 37.5 mmol (1500 mg) in later life, but the value of a high intake is unproven (see NIH Consensus, 1984). Vitamin D deficiency should be avoided by adequate exposure to sunlight (or if necessary by dietary supplements of calciferol 12.5 µg/day) because low grade osteomalacia may also predispose to fracture of the hip.

Rickets and osteomalacia

The requirements for vitamin D are met largely from exposure of the skin to ultraviolet light. The average diet contains a mean of 2–3 µg calciferol/day (fortified margarine, eggs and fatty fish are the chief sources) whereas human needs are four times this amount. Rickets is now a rare condition in the UK except in the Asian community. The high extraction flour used in chappati appears to accelerate the breakdown of cholecalciferol. In addition Asian children may produce less cholecalciferol in the skin than most of their British counterparts. Rickets may also occur in patients with malabsorption or renal disease and in epileptics taking anticonvulsant drugs.

Osteomalacia of mild degree is also probably quite common in elderly infirm subjects. If liver pathology can be excluded, a raised serum alkaline phosphatase is the best screening test for osteomalacia (false negatives <15%); measurement of isoenzymes is also helpful. Bone scanning with radiolabelled diphosphonate may be used to confirm the diagnosis as well as to exclude causes for a raised bone alkaline phosphatase such as metastases and Paget's disease.

Recognition and Management of Nutritional Disorders

Patients with uncomplicated vitamin D deficiency should be given 25–50 μg calciferol per day (1000–2000 IU). This is sufficient to heal the nutritional bone lesion in all age groups. It will also be effective in patients with mild–moderate malabsorption but not in those with severe malabsorption or a renal lesion affecting vitamin D metabolism. It may be given for at least 3 months without risk of causing hypervitaminosis D.

Elderly house-bound people taking a diet containing little vitamin D should be given calciferol in a dose equivalent to 12.5 μg (1500 IU)/day. The incidence of D-deficient myopathy in the elderly is unknown but persistant low-grade osteomalacia predisposes to hip fractures. In treating patients for deficiency of vitamin D it is necessary to ensure that the intake of calcium is adequate (at least 1 g/day) (Table 4.2) and

Table 4.2 *The calcium content of foods*

Calcium content of some common foods

Milk (1 pint, 570 ml)	650 mg
Cheese-hard (2 oz, 56 g)	300 mg (variable)
Bread (fortified) (4 oz, 112 g)	120 mg
Vegetables (4 oz, 112 g)	30 mg
Egg (standard)	20 mg
Potato (4 oz, 112 g)	10 mg

Milk and cheese are by far the best sources of calcium in the British diet. If bread were not fortified the intake of many adults would fall to 300 mg or less calcium per day. In hard water areas moderate amounts of calcium are ingested inadvertently. (The concentration of calcium in water may reach 30 mg/100 ml.)

if necessary to supplement the diet with an appropriate pharmacological preparation of calcium (e.g. effervescent calcium tablets each containing 400 mg calcium).

NUTRITIONAL DEFICIENCIES IN ALCOHOLICS

A high intake of alcohol (which provides 7 kcal (29 kJ) energy/g) is often associated with poor dietary habits. Thus some degree of malnutrition is common in alcoholics, especially among those who are poor (skid-row alcoholics). Moreover, alcohol interferes with the absorption of some nutrients (e.g. thiamine), may increase the requirements (e.g. of folic acid) or the excretion of others (e.g. magnesium) and may alter intermediary metabolism (e.g. by predisposing susceptible individuals to hyperlipidaemia).

It is often difficult to distinguish between the toxic effects of alcohol and the results of malnutrition. For example red cell macrocytosis occurs in 90% of subjects drinking more than 80 g alcohol per day. Folate and pyridoxine deficiency are common and may contribute to the disturbed haematopoesis. On the other hand, alcohol has a direct effect on the bone marrow and in most cases this appears to be the main cause of the macrocytosis. Similarly, the heart may be affected by thiamine deficiency (beri-beri heart disease) and by the direct effects of alcohol (alcoholic cardiomyopathy).

Excess alcohol may adversely affect the function of every body system. The interactions between the direct toxic effects of alcohol and the secondary effects of malnutrition are seen especially well in the pancreas and the liver. Pancreatitis occurs in about 30% of alcoholics and is both caused by and contributes to nutritional deficiency. Liver disease is just as prevalent. Again nutritional deficiency may predispose to liver damage. Conversely changes in hepatic metabolism may lead to a type IV hyperlipidaemia (alcohol- and carbohydrate-induced hypertriglyceridaemia) and to both hypo- and hyperglycaemia.

Nutritional deficiencies found in alcoholics are listed in Table 4.3. Vitamin B deficiency is an important consideration. All chronic alcoholics ill enough to require admission to hospital should be given a vitamin B preparation intravenously. Wernicke's encephalopathy (a rare condition in general hospital practice) may be missed in the patient who is believed to be suffering from the direct toxic effects of alcohol, from delerium tremens, or from the effects of alcohol-associated cerebral atrophy. In addition, serious metabolic disturbances may be revealed by a full metabolic profile, especially in the binge drinker. These include hypokalaemia, hypomagnesaemia, hypophosphataemia, hypoglycaemia and disturbed acid-base balance, e.g. metabolic alkalosis (from vomiting) and alcoholic ketoacidosis.

MALNUTRITION IN SUBJECTS TAKING SPECIFIC DIETS

The taking of a mixed diet (see p. 9) protects the normal person against nutritional disturbances. Limited diets carry the risk of specific deficiencies (Table 4.4).

Table 4.3 Nutritional deficiencies occurring in alcoholics

Deficient nutrient	Effect
Protein	Fatty liver*
	Muscle wasting*
Vitamins	
B group	Beri—beri heart disease
	Wernicke—Korsakoff syndrome
	Peripheral neuropathy*
Vitamin B6	Sideroblastic erthroblastosis
Folic acid	Megaloblastic anaemia
Minerals and trace elements	
Phosphate	Hypophosphataemia
Magnesium	Hypomagnesaemia—Tetany, fits, dysrhythmias
Zinc	Hypozincaemia—?effect

*Direct organ damage by alcohol complicates the clinical picture.

Table 4.4 Nutritional deficiencies caused by limited diets

Type of diet	Nature of diet	Potential deficiencies

Zen macrobiotic	Diet graded through self-deprivation. May be severely limited (often only cereal group)	Vitamins, especially Vitamin A and D
		Folic acid
		Ascorbic acid
		Minerals
		  Calcium
		  Iron

'Junk' food	Processed foods high in fat, sugar (and often salt)	Fibre Zinc (may predispose to obesity)
Food faddism	Often associated with 'intolerance' especially to wheat, eggs and dairy products	Rarely taken to extremes but care should be taken with subjects on severely limited diets
Asian diets	High phytate interferes with calcium/vitamin D metabolism	May predispose to osteomalacia
Low calorie 'complete' liquid diets in treatment of obesity	300–400 kcal (1250–1700 kJ) 40–50 g protein/day. Vitamins and trace elements at recommended daily allowance (RDA) levels	Promote rapid weight loss. Useful in patients with severe obesity but should be used with care. Body protein is lost ? effect

For example a small but increasing number of people are attracted to vegetarian diets. These are deemed 'healthy' because in general they are high in fibre and low in saturated fat and cholesterol. On the other hand many plant proteins are incomplete. They lack one or more essential amino acids. The problem is easily overcome if the subject takes dairy products, eggs or fish regularly. A strict vegetarian (vegan) should eat as wide a range of food stuffs as possible. Nuts and cereal grains contain limited amounts of lysine and isoleucine. This can be balanced by a good intake of leafy vegetables and roots (which are poor sources of methionine) and of legumes (deficient of tryptophan). In addition a vegetarian diet tends to be low in calcium and riboflavin unless there is a liberal intake of dark green leafy vegetables. A vegan diet contains little vitamin D and no vitamin B12. Many vegetarians take fortified soy milk to guard against potential deficiencies.

DRUGS PREDISPOSING TO NUTRIENT DEFICIENCIES

Drugs and nutrients interact in three important ways:

1. Nutrient intake may affect enzymes which metabolize drugs, e.g. in the severely malnourished antibiotics are more slowly metabolized.
2. Drugs may increase the requirements for nutrients by affecting appetite, absorption and intermediary metabolism.
3. Nutrients in large amounts may decrease or increase the toxicity of drugs, e.g. the use of cysteine or methionine in paracetamol poisoning.

Clinicians must be aware of these interactions. In this chapter we are concerned particularly with drugs which may alter nutritional status. Many drugs impair appetite including: antibiotics (e.g. ampicillin, streptomycin, tetracycline, metronidazole); the anticoagulant, phenindione; the antihistamine, chlorpheniramine; some antihypertensive agents, e.g. captopril, diazoxide, hydrallazine; the cholesterol lowering agent, clofibrate; most cytotoxic agents and some psychoactive drugs (lithium, phenytoin). Examples of drugs which affect absorption and metabolism are listed in Table 4.5.

Table 4.5 Effects of some drugs on nutrition

Drug group	Effect	Significance
Antacids	May contain excessive Na Chelate phosphate (Al Mg Ca)	Fluid retention Hypophosphataemia

Antibiotics	Bile salt binding (Neomycin)
	Metabolic effects
	    Isoniazid
	
	    Pyrimethamine
	    Trimethoprim
	    Amphotericin
		Fat malabsorption
		
		Increases requirements of vitamin B6
		
		Increases requirements of folate
		
		Hypomagnesaemia

Anticonvulsants	Intermediate metabolism
	    Phenobarbitone
	    Phenytoin
		Increases requirements of folate and vitamins B12 and D

Chelating agents	Bind bile salts (cholestyramine)	Fat malabsorption
Contraceptive pill	Alter Folate and B6 metabolism	? significance
Corticosteroids	Increase appetite Increase protein catabolism Decrease Ca transport Decrease CHO tolerance Retention salt and water	Weight gain Muscle wasting Osteoporosis Hyperglycaemia Increase BP Hypokalaemia
Cytotoxic drugs	Inhibit appetite Antagonise folate metabolism	Weight loss Folate deficiency
Diuretics	Increase excretion electrolytes	Hypokalaemia Hypomagnesaemia
L-Dopa	B6 antagonist	Increases requirements of vitamin B6
Mefenamic acid	Mucosal damage	Diarrhoea Weight loss
NSAID	Prostaglandin synthetase inhibitor (increase intestinal permeability)	Occasionally diarrhoea

OBESITY

Obesity is the most common nutritional disorder in the Western World. But clinicians find the condition difficult to define precisely and for the most part impossible to manage satisfactorily. Data correlating weight with indices of health are far from ideal. Several methods have been used to define obesity. The most commonly used is derived from calculations of Quetelet's Index (Table 4.6). If American Metropolitan Life Insurance figures are used, an ideal weight for young adults is given by an index of 20 to 25. Applying these figures to the UK might suggest that half the population is overweight. On the other hand mortality data from a variety of sources shows little or no evidence of excess mortality for the lesser degrees of obesity (Fig. 4.4). A better definition of risk may be obtained from assessments of the distribution of body fat from measurements of waist and hip circumferences. The risk for ischaemic heart disease and stroke rises steeply with waist–hip ratios of greater than 1.0 for men and 0.8 for women.

In a general practice covering a population of 2500, one person may be grossly obese (W/H^2 = >40), 5–10 obese (W/H^2 = 35–40) and a further 80–100 seriously overweight (W/H^2 = 30–35). The side-effects of obesity are considerable (see Table 4.8). The concern of those afflicted is reflected in the millions of pounds spent each year on magazines, books, diets and exercise programmes which claim to show how to lose weight effectively. In the short term almost any rational approach to weight loss is effective but less than 10% of those treated will succeed in maintaining a satisfactory lower weight for more than a year. Faced with these facts many practitioners are nihilistic. They take the view, either that severe obesity is a form of original sin which the afflicted deserve to suffer, or that it is a metabolic disorder of unknown cause which is essentially untreatable. In fact the management of an obese subject presents the clinician with an interesting challenge.

Before considering how best to meet this challenge some basic observations need to be emphasized:

1. Genes are important in determining body weight. The prevalence of obesity amongst children of slim parents is less than 10%, with one obese parent the figure rises to 40% and with both parents obese it exceeds 66%.
2. Environment is of lesser importance. Indeed a recent study of 540 Danish adoptees showed a strong correlation between weight class of adoptees and body mass index of natural parents (mothers <0.0001, fathers <0.02) but not with that of adoptive parents.

Table 4.6 Definition of Obesity

$$\text{Quetelet's Index} = \frac{\text{Weight in kg}}{(\text{Height in m})^2}$$

20–25	Grade 0	Ideal weight range
25–30	Grade 1	Overweight
30–40	Grade 2	Moderately obese
Over 40	Grade 3	Grossly obese

3. Overfeeding in infancy is not an important predisposing cause. The hypothesis that infant feeding determines the number of fat cells in the body and controls the tendency to obesity rests on an insecure basis.
4. Overt endocrine disease is rarely a cause of obesity.
5. The obese have a range of basal metabolic rates consistent with their muscle mass and in this respect they are not fundamentally different from the lean.
6. The behaviour of an obese person to food may be different from that of the non-obese. In particular, there is some evidence to suggest a more rapid response to external cues for feeding, such as time of day, sight, smell and taste of food, and advertisements. In contrast the response to internal stimuli of satiety appears much less readily.
7. The effect of overfeeding may also be different in the obese compared with the lean; although the evidence in this respect is difficult to interpret.

Management of the overweight (mild–moderate obesity)

Most overweight subjects are no more than 10 kg overweight. It is quite impractical for doctors to be directly involved in the management of all in this group who wish to lose weight. Fortunately this is rarely required. In most areas the problem is covered more than adequately by community health programmes and responsible commercial slimming organizations.

The clinician's role is primarily one of excluding causative or associated pathology, of sensing the need of the patient to lose weight and of providing information on available facilities. With the aid of dietitians many GPs have started slimming groups. Most of these

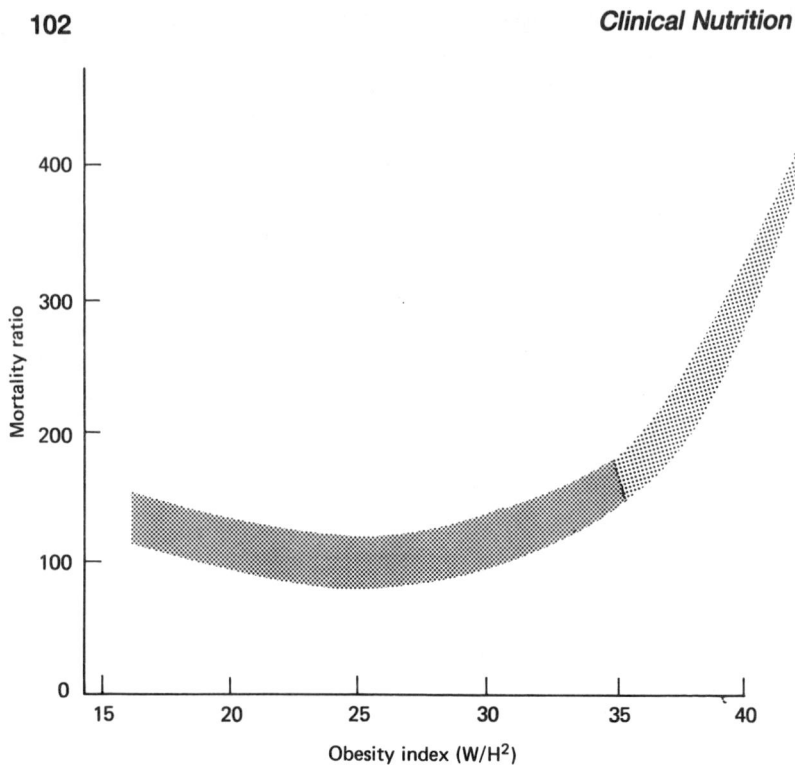

Figure 4.4 Relation of obesity index to mortality. (Graph modified from:

Seltzer C. C. (1966). Some re-evaluation of the build and blood pressure study 1959 as related to pondiral index, somatotype and mortality. *New Engl. J. Med*; **274**: 254–9.

The modification takes into account more recent data, e.g.:

Keys A. (1980). Overweight, obesity, coronary heart disease and mortality. *Nutr. Rev*; **38**: 297–307. Sorlie P., Gordon T., Kannel W. B. (1980). Body build and mortality. The Framingham study. *J.A.M.A*; **243**: 1828–31.)

Note that minimal mortality appears to be associated with grade 0–1 (W/H^2 20–30) obesity and that there is a distinct increase in mortality ratios of underweight individuals (in part due to smoking) and that the data on the increased mortality ratios of the very obese is unsatisfactory.

groups run on a self-help basis with relatively little professional input. Nevertheless the results of their efforts may depend on medical attitudes. With enthusiastic practitioners it is possible to increase public awareness of means of improving health and well-being. Many

Recognition and Management of Nutritional Disorders 103

Coronary Prevention Studies have demonstrated a prolonged change in the attitudes of participants. They lose weight, reduce their levels of circulating cholesterol, reduce cigarette smoking and increase their fitness by exercise and maintain these changes over several years.

The general practitioner can help by identifying those at risk, especially young people who are starting to gain weight, by weighing patients regularly and by keeping a record of the progress of those who are striving to lose excess fat.

Most people treat the doctor's opinion with great respect. The doctor can make use of this privileged position to good effect. He will know the family circumstances, the stresses and strains of life and the difficulties of dietary control for certain groups in the practice, particularly young mothers. Management of family problems may be invaluable in helping people apply the self-discipline needed to lose weight effectively. It is also helpful to assess the normal eating habits and dietary patterns of overweight subjects. A modest degree of weight loss can be achieved by following simple dietetic principles. (Table 4.7).

Management of the grossly obese subject

The management of the grossly obese person presents the clinician with a much more difficult problem. Insurance statistics show a mortality rate which increases with the degree of obesity. There is little or no effect with modest overweight (Quetelet's Index 25–30) but as the Index moves from 30 to 35 the expected mortality increases 50% (see Fig. 4.4). Above these levels there appears to be a rapid increase in mortality ratios but the available data is limited because the very obese are usually unable to obtain life insurance.

The complications of obesity are listed in Table 4.8. Thus both morbidity and mortality are increased in the obese. It is much less certain, however, that the excess weight causes the additional morbidity. Moreover there are no satisfactory clinical trials to show that weight loss can prevent or correct the disorders listed. Nevertheless, the circumstantial evidence is favourable. Patients and the lay public have little doubt about the benefits; and in one important study subjects who were refused insurance at normal premiums on account of obesity and who subsequently achieved a normal weight were shown to have a mortality record comparable to that of people who were never overweight.

Table 4.7 *Treatment of mild obesity*

1. Dietary Advice
    Calorie counting (using food tables)—This is tedious and suitable for a few obsessional subjects
    Food categorisation into free foods, forbidden and restricted (see below). Acceptable especially to men
    Low carbohydrate—avoidance virtually all carbohydrate foods. Acceptable especially to women
2. Regular weighing and encouragement
    General Practitioner groups
    Dietitian groups (usually Health Centre based)
    Commercial slimming clubs
3. Exercise programmes
    Adapted to individual preferences
    Aim to increase fitness (effect on weight may be minimal)

Food categories

Free foods	Restricted foods	Forbidden foods
Meat	Bread	Sugar and
Eggs	Butter/margarine	sweet foods
Fish	Cereals	Cakes, biscuits
Salads	Milk	and pastries
Vegetables	Cheese	Rice
Potatoes		Pastas
(boiled or baked)		Ice cream
Fresh fruit		Alcohol

There is, of course, no absolute definition of severe obesity. The distribution of values obtained from a general population gives an open J-shaped curve which makes cut-off points on the ascending limb quite arbitrary (see Fig. 4.4).

Nevertheless, an Index of 35 indicates an excess weight of well over 30 kg (or over 5 stones). For a man of average height this means a weight of 110 kg (18 stones) and for a woman 90 kg (over 14 stones). Even a most determined person will take at least a year to lose this amount of excess weight by dietary means.

Professional help is needed and at present this may be best given from a hospital clinic. It is necessary to:

Table 4.8 Effects of obesity and the potential benefit of weight loss

Findings in the obese	Results of weight loss
Metabolic changes	
Reduced glucose tolerance	Markedly improves
Increased plasma triglycerides, cholesterol, uric acid	Improves
Increased prevalence of pathology	
Diabetes mellitus	Better control
Hypertension—Vascular disease	Some improvement
Gall bladder disease	No effect
Fatty liver	May resolve
Osteoarthritis	
Gout	Symptomatic improvement
Herniae	
Varicose veins	
Intertriginous dermatitis	
Exercise intolerance	Considerable improvement
Social disability	Often lessens

Table 4.9 Metabolic assessment of the obese patient

Age, sex
Body composition (fat:muscle)
Excess body calories (excess weight (kg) × 7000) = X kcal
Resting metabolic rate
Calories required to maintain weight = C kcal/day
Calories in proposed diet = D kcal/day
Time needed to shed excess calories = X/C−D days*

*This is a minimal estimate as the value of C will fall as weight decreases.

1. Determine the nature and degree of obesity. Estimate approximate calorie excess (Table 4.9).
2. Exclude causative organic disease (e.g. Cushing's syndrome), even though an underlying physical disorder is very unlikely.
3. Assess associated pathology (e.g. diabetes mellitus) and determine whether or not there is physical disability or psychological maladjustment.

4. Undertake a psychosocial assessment in order to try to determine an appropriate strategy (Table 4.10).
5. Decide a form of management and set realistic objectives.

Table 4.10 *Assessment of attitudes of the obese subject*

Factors contributing to weight gain
Results of previous efforts to lose weight
Rate of weight loss patient believes possible
Expectations of effects of weight loss
Social class and educational achievements
Drive and determination
Psychosocial history
Drugs (including alcohol and tobacco)

The management of an obese young, mildly hypertensive but otherwise fit man with a bad family history of coronary artery disease who has recently married, presents a completely different problem from that of an obese postmenopausal sedentary woman prone to depression who lives on her own in a small village. Both need medical help and support but the objectives are quite different.

The potential gain for the young man is considerable. He is muscular and will have a high resting metabolic rate. For a given caloric deficit he will lose weight considerably more quickly than the middle-aged woman. He is likely to be well-motivated and it should be possible to enlist the help of his wife. The dietary regimen should be designed to reduce the level of circulating lipids (especially low-density lipoprotein – cholesterol) as well as leading to significant loss of weight. Exercise may play an important part in the overall programme. If necessary extreme measures may be indicated (Table 4.11).

In contrast, the objectives for the postmenopausal woman will be much more limited. Massive weight loss is unrealistic. This patient takes little physical exercise and has a small lean body mass. Her metabolic requirements may be considerably less than 1500 kcals (6.7 MJ) per day. If she can be persuaded to reduce her intake by a third, her weight loss may be no more than 1–2 kg a month. But an overall loss of 10 kg may be enough to relieve the pain in her osteoarthritic hips and to improve her self-image. Successful management will include her

Table 4.11 Possible modes of treatment of severely obese subjects $(W/H^2>35)$

Strict reducing diet—weigh all food (circa 800 kcal (3300 kJ))
Milk diet with added iron, vitamins and, if necessary, fibre (400–600 kcal (1650–2500 kJ))
Drugs to reduce appetite (e.g. diethylpropion) and enhance satiety (e.g. fenfluramine)
Wire jaws
Semistarvation (in-patient care)
Gastric balloon
Surgery (at present gastric stapling is the method of choice)

acceptance of her body as it is. This will be easier if her appearance can be improved by skilled counselling and by the help of ancillary services.

A sequence of possible treatments is outlined in Table 4.11. The way in which these treatments are applied depends on the judgement of the clinician and the dietician's skill in providing a diet which the patient can manage. Liquid diets carry the advantage that the patient cannot cheat unknowingly but sooner or later most subjects find this form of nutrition intolerably monotonous. Jaw wiring is often extraordinarily effective in holding down caloric intake for several months but most subjects relapse badly after their jaws are released. Some authorities fasten a nylon cord around the waist of the patient who has lost much weight after successful dieting with or without jaw wiring. This acts as a permanent reminder of the new body image and as a psychological crutch.

Surgery is a last resort which is much more popular in the USA than in Europe. Stapling the stomach to reduce it to a hopper with carefully measured volume of no more than 60 ml and an outlet of 12 mm (banded with a ring of non-absorbable material) appears to be the most satisfactory procedure. Most patients lose weight satisfactorily but they pay a high price. They are rendered permanently unable to eat a normal meal. Attempts to do so lead to vomiting. Relatively few patients believe the rewards of weight loss are sufficient to balance the risks of surgery and its inevitable side-effects. Nevertheless, the carefully selected patient may do very well. Careful follow-up should be given to such a patient after surgery. Good dietary advice is needed in order to avoid the malnutrition which may occur with a self-restricted diet.

Drugs

Drugs play little part in the management of obesity. They may be used to suppress appetite. Amphetamine and related drugs (e.g. diethylpropion) appear to reduce hunger by acting on catecholamine neurotransmitters. Fenfluramine enhances satiety through its interactions with serotonin. These drugs also have an effect on intermediary metabolism. They may provide some short-term benefit but they appear to do no more than to make dieting tolerable. They do not help establish new eating habits. Diethylpropion may be used for a few weeks at a time in order to help the patient over a difficult stage; fenfluramine must be used more careully because of its side-effects on the central nervous system (sudden stopping of fenfluramine may cause depression). Some authorities favour the long-term use of drugs but the results are not very impressive. All clinicians agree that weight gain occurs rapidly on stopping treatment.

The use of drugs to increase energy losses is equally unsatisfactory. Thyroid hormone has been given to prevent the decrease in metabolic rate associated with weight loss. This increases the proportion of nitrogen lost as weight decreases, may damage cardiac muscle and alters the function of the thyroid gland. The long-term results of giving thyroxine to euthyroid obese patients are no better than treatment with diet alone.

Whichever form of treatment is used the clinician must be realistic about the rather poor chances of success measured in terms of weight loss. Considerably less than half his patients with severe obesity ($W/H^2 > 35$) will do really well. Yet nearly all will be openly grateful for the attention of their doctor even if they lose little weight. Often the obese subject is unable to tolerate a strict diet. The 'failure' needs help and sympathy much more often than scolding. Success should not be measured solely in terms of weight loss. The patient who has learned something of his own physiology and of himself in relation to his environment may have achieved more than the clinician realizes.

HYPERLIPIDAEMIA

Hyperlipidaemia is a common condition and a case can be made for routine screening in young adults (Table 4.12). It should be standard practice to measure circulating lipids in patients with premature

Table 4.12 Laboratory values for circulating lipids

	Cholesterol	Triglycerides
Normal	3.6–6.0 mmol/l (140–240 mg/dl)	M. 0.7–2.1 mmol/l (65–190 mg/dl) F. 0.6–1.5 mmol/l (55–135 mg/dl)
Mild elevation	Up to 7.5 mmol/l (300 mg/dl)	Up to 3.3 mmol/l (300 mg/dl)
Marked elevation	More than 7.5 mmol/l	More than 3.3 mmol/l

atheromatous disease, with gout, with xanthomata, or with corneal arcus at an early age. Relatives of those with a genetically-determined form of hyperlipidaemia should be offered investigation.

The clinician must attempt to classify the disorder (Table 4.13) and to offer appropriate treatment. Types II and IV are the common disorders. Type II hypercholesterolaemia is strongly associated with premature coronary artery disease. The genetic form of type IIa is characterized by a reduced clearance of low-density lipoproteins (LDL) because of a lack of cellular receptors. Homozygotes for the condition have very high values of circulating cholesterol and often die in early adolescence. Heterozygotes vary considerably. Severely affected males have coronary artery disease in early adult life; less severely affected subjects may reach middle age without difficulty, especially if they are female.

Without a family history it is difficult to separate patients with genetically-determined heterozygous hypercholesterolaemia from subjects at the upper end of the normal range for circulating cholesterol (which may be determined, at least in part, by diet). A similar pattern of hyperlipidaemia may occur as a result of other pathologies but very low-density lipoprotein (VLDL) is usually increased as well as LDL (type IIb 'common mixed hyperlipidaemia'). Type IV hyperlipidaemia is nearly always related to diet (high refined carbohydrate, excess alcohol) and may be secondary to a variety of disorders especially obesity, uncontrolled diabetes and alcohol abuse. It may cause gout, eruptive xanthomata and possibly premature atheroma.

Most patients with hyperlipidaemia require dietary advice as well as treatment of associated clinical disorders (Table 4.13). Those with mild hyperlipidaemia can be managed by dietary means alone. Subjects with type IIa hyperlipidaemia are advised to eat a low cholesterol, high

Table 4.13 *The hyperlipidaemias*

Type	Frequency	Causes	Clinical manifestations	Laboratory findings	Treatment

I	Very rare	Genetic
		Secondary
		  Diabetes
		  Pancreatitis
		  Dysproteinaemia
			Abdominal pain
			Pancreatitis
			Eruptive xanthomata
				Creamy plasma
				Chylomicronaemia
				Triglycerides +++
					Low fat diet

IIa	Prevalence 0.5%
	(Homozygotes rare <1:1000)
		Genetic
		Primary—?
		  diet-induced
		Secondary
		e.g. Myxoedema
		  Obstructive jaundice
		  Nephrosis
			Early atheroma
			Corneal arcus
			Tendinous and tuberous xanthoma
				Clear serum
				LDL ++
				Cholesterol ++
				TG normal
					Low saturated fat diet
					Low cholesterol
					Cholestyramine
					(Nicotinic acid)

IIb	Quite common	Nearly always secondary (as IIa)	As for IIa	Usually clear serum LDL and VLDL ++ Cholesterol and TG ++	As above Also low refined CHO No alcohol (Clofibrate)

III	Uncommon	Rarely genetic
		Secondary
		  Uncontrolled diabetes
		  Myxoedema
			Diabetic with early atheroma
			Arcus
			Xanthomata
				Usually turbid serum
				IDL ++
				Cholesterol and TG ++
					As for IIb

Table 4.13 The hyperlipidaemias

Type	Frequency	Causes	Clinical manifestations	Laboratory findings	Treatment
IV	Common	Rarely genetic Primary diet-induced Secondary e.g. Uncontrolled diabetes Alcohol abuse Renal dialysis Pancreatitis	Diabetes Obesity Gout Occasionally eruptive xanthoma	Often turbid serum VLDL ++ Cholesterol usually normal TG +++	Low refined carbohydrate No alcohol Weight reduction
V	Uncommon	Rarely genetic Secondary Uncontrolled diabetes Alcohol Pancreatitis Steroids	Obese diabetic Abdominal pain Pancreatitis Gout Eruptive xanthoma Sensory neuropathy	Serum turbid Chylomicronaemia VLDL +++ Cholesterol often +	Low fat/refined CHO No alcohol Clofibrate (Nicotinic acid)

polyunsaturated fat diet with added fibre. This will reduce cholesterol levels by 10–20%. Mild hyperlipidaemia in patients with a type IV pattern responds to reducing diets with restricted carbohydrate and if necessary abstinence from alcohol.

More severely affected patients require treatment with drugs to lower the concentration of circulating lipids. This is particularly important for young males, especially if they have a family history of hyperlipidaemia. Each case must be considered on its merits. The available drugs have important side-effects and there are a few data to show that their long-term use is both safe and effective. In practice, the patient should be established on a diet before being offered the drugs. These should then be introduced one at a time and the efficacy of each preparation assessed by careful follow up (Table 4.14).

Table 4.14 *Drugs used in the treatment of the hyperlipidaemias*

Drug	Dose	Action
Cholestyramine	8–16 g b.d.	Sequesters bile acids Accelerates LDL clearance
Clofibrate	500 mg b.d.	Decreases VLDL Accelerates VLDL–LDL Reduces hepatic synthesis of cholesterol
Nicotinic acid	1–3 g t.d.s.	Decreases LDL and IDL Inhibits lipolysis Inhibits production VLDL

DIET IN THE MANAGEMENT OF SPECIFIC DISEASE

Diabetes mellitus

Diet has always been important in the management of diabetes mellitus. Before the discovery of insulin patients were starved of carbohydrate in order to try to prolong life. Today the dietary manipulations are more subtle. The nutritionist aims to minimize

Table 4.15 *The glycaemic index*

Comparison of rise in blood sugar induced by foods containing equivalent amounts of carbohydrates

Food	%
Glucose	100%
Honey Mashed white potato	90%
White bread Rice New potatoes	70%
Mars bar Wholemeal bread Brown rice Shredded wheat	60%
Sugar Pastry White spaghetti All-bran Yams	50%
Whole meal spaghetti Sweet potatoes Peas	40%
Butter beans Ice cream Tomato soup	30%
Kidney beans Lentils	20%
Fructose Soya beans Peanuts	10%

glycaemia (Table 4.15) to avoid large swings in the levels of blood sugar and to control the tendency to hyperlipidaemia. The patient's life-style, requirements for insulin or oral hypoglycaemic agents and the complications of the diabetic process must be taken into account. Here we are concerned solely with guidelines for dietary manipulation.

The achievement of a desirable body weight is the first objective (see Table 3.2). Usually this means reducing overall caloric intake primarily by avoiding energy-dense foods (simple carbohydrates and fats). Swings in blood sugar may be minimized by taking a diet comprising 50% complex carbohydrates, 30% fat and 20% protein. In essence, such a diet allows an unrestricted intake of vegetables, unrefined starches and fresh fruit, protein foods low in fat, such as lean meat, chicken, white fish, skimmed milk and cottage cheese, and appropriate amounts of fat depending on the overall allowance of calories. In insulin-dependent diabetics the diet should be distributed through the day in relation to the requirements for insulin. Finally it is important to remember that diabetic patients are prone to hyperlipidaemia and to premature atheroma. Dietary guidelines should include advice regarding the intake of cholesterol and of the ratio of saturated to polyunsaturated fatty acids (see p. 109).

Gastrointestinal disease

In the UK most clinicians with an interest in clinical nutrition also specialize in gastroenterology. This reflects the high incidence of nutritional disorders associated with gastrointestinal disease (Table 4.16). Conversely malnutrition may cause gastrointestinal disease.

Table 4.16 Specific nutrient deficiencies associated with malabsorptive disorders

Disorder	Deficiency
Gastric surgery	Iron Vitamin B12 (after many years) Calcium and vitamin D
Coeliac disease	Iron (zinc) Folic acid
Tropical sprue	Folic acid Vitamin B12 (after many years)
Crohn's disease	Iron (from blood loss) Folic acid (Zinc)
Massive resection small intestine	Most nutrients including electrolytes Magnesium deficiency common Essential fatty acid deficiency

This is seen particularly in the mouth. Angular stomatitis, glossitis and periodontal disease are sometimes diet-related (see p. 70).

Teeth

The high intake of refined carbohydrate in the developed world (especially of sucrose) predisposes children to dental caries. Nevertheless other factors, particularly the amount of fluoride ingested, are clearly important as shown by the dramatic fall in the incidence of caries over the past decade (see Fig. 6.2, p. 185).

The oesophagus

Oesophageal disorders may cause dysphagia. Weight loss is common and supplementary nutrition is often necessary either via a soft nasogastric tube or via an enterostomy. In some cases total parenteral nutrition may be more appropriate. Improving the nutritional status of patients before major oesophageal surgery has been found to reduce postoperative morbidity. Gastro-oesophageal reflux leads to oesophagitis with heartburn, bleeding and sometimes stricture formation. Patients with symptoms of reflux should be encouraged to eat small regular frequent meals so that the stomach does not get overdistended; to avoid spirits, hot drinks and spicy foods which may damage the inflamed oesophagus; to limit the intake of fat; to avoid methylxanthine-containing beverages and alcohol which encourage reflux by reducing lower oesophageal sphincter pressure; to take antacids to relieve symptoms, and if obese, to lose weight. In severely affected patients H2-receptor antagonists may be used to suppress gastric acid secretion, and metoclopramide to encourage gastric emptying and to enhance the tone of the lower oesophageal sphincter. Omeprazole has been shown to be effective in treating oesophagitis in patients resistant to all other forms of treatment but this drug has not yet been released for general use.

The stomach

The stomach acts as a reservoir for ingested food. It secretes pepsin and acid which are mixed with the masticated boluses of food received from the oesophagus to produce chyme. The release of chyme into the duodenum is carefully regulated and thus intestinal function may be disturbed after any form of gastric surgery. The relationship of diet to gastric pathology has not been clearly established. Alcohol and possibly highly-spiced foods may cause gastritis. It has also been suggested that poor nutrition predisposes to gastric ulceration, but the evidence is only circumstantial. (In the UK, between the wars, gastric ulcer was much more prevalent in the poorly-fed lower social classes.) Strict diets are no longer used in the treatment of peptic ulceration. Indeed the Sippy regimen of hourly milk and frequent antacids may have caused as much harm from hypercalcaemia, hypercalciuria and alkalosis ('milk-alkali' syndrome) as good. Diet is used simply to reduce dyspeptic symptoms. Patients are advised to take small frequent regular meals, to avoid alcohol (which stimulates acid secretion) and mucosal irritants, such as spicy foods and non-steroidal anti-inflammatory drugs.

Postgastric surgery

Early problems. Dumping occurs in up to 20% of patients after gastric surgery. It appears to be caused by the rapid passage of hypertonic nutrients into the small intestine. Extracellular fluid pouring into the lumen of the gut reduces plasma volume and causes the symptoms of 'early dumping'. Rapid absorption of carbohydrate leads to hyperglycaemia which in turn stimulates the secretion of insulin and causes a rapid fall in the level of blood sugar – 'late dumping'.

Symptoms occur more commonly in women than in men, in those with a gastroenterostomy rather than a pyloroplasty and in patients who have had a total rather than selective vagotomy.

The aim of treatment is to reduce the osmolarity of the intestinal contents and to prolong the emptying time of the gastric remnant. Meals should be small and taken dry, the diet should contain little refined carbohydrate, drinks should be taken separately from the main meal and the patient may find it helpful to lie down after eating. Occasionally the symptoms of reactive hypoglycaemia can be relieved by taking tolbutamide with meals.

Rapid gastric emptying also predisposes to diarrhoea. Altered neurohormonal control of intestinal transit and spill-over of bile acids into the colon increase colonic contents and promote rapid emptying of the bowel. Symptoms usually settle if the diet is modified as for the dumping syndrome. Occasionally symptoms are sufficiently severe to consider using a bile-sequestering agent (e.g. cholestyramine).

After gastric surgery it is also wise to advise the patient of the dangers of swallowing poorly masticated undigestable food materials, such as orange pith. Such material may obstruct the small intestine.

Late problems. Weight loss is common after gastric surgery, especially after extensive gastrectomy for cancer of the stomach. Women find it more difficult to adapt than men. Nevertheless, severe protein-energy malnutrition is uncommon and usually indicates associated pathology. Hypoproteinaemia is never due solely to the effects of uncomplicated gastric surgery. It may be caused by associated intestinal pathology such as coeliac disease, stagnant loop syndrome or chronic pancreatitis.

Specific nutrient deficiencies are common 5 or more years after gastric resection. Patients should be checked annually. The correction of specific deficiencies often leads to an improved appetite and a general improvement in well-being (Table 4.16).

Small intestine

The final stages of digestion occur within the small intestine, which is also responsible for the absorption of most nutrients (Fig. 4.5). Failure of these functions is the most common reason for total parenteral nutrition.

Normally most carbohydrate, protein, water-soluble vitamins, minerals and fluid are absorbed in the upper small intestine. The duodenum is particularly important for the absorption of divalent cations (especially iron and calcium). Fat and fat-soluble vitamins may spill over into the ileum which also has specific receptors for the absorption of bile salts and vitamin B12. The ileum absorbs water and salt efficiently and has an important chloride–bicarbonate exchange mechanism. It is estimated that 1–1.5 l of fluid a day pass through the ileocaecal valve into the colon carrying 100—150 mmol sodium and perhaps 2–6% of unabsorbed nutrients.

The small intestine has considerable reserve capacity and is capable of adapting to localized pathology. The ileum can take over all functions of the jejunum and thus resection of a metre or more of jejunum has little or no long-term adverse effects. Coeliac disease affects primarily the duodenum and upper jejunum. Many patients have no diarrhoea or steatorrhoea although deficiencies of iron and folic acid are common. In part, this reflects the importance of duodenal function. Loss of short lengths of ileum are also tolerated well because

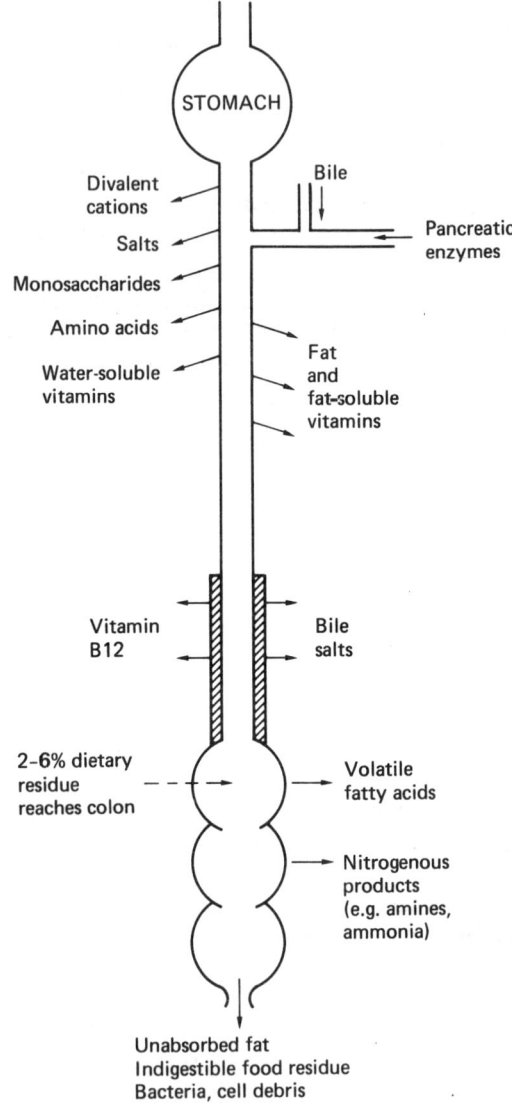

Figure 4.5 Sites of absorption of nutrients from the small intestine (diagram modified from Fig. 10, p. 1524 by kind permission from Booth C. C. (1968). In *Handbook of Physiology*, Section 6, Vol. 3. Washington D.C: American Physiological Society.)

the colon has reserve capacity. But removal of all the ileum or loss of the ileocaecal valve nearly always results in persistent diarrhoea. Diet is important in the long-term management of chronic disorders of the small intestine. Some details are summarized in Table 4.17.

Table 4.17 Diets for patients with small intestinal disease

Disorder	Diet	Comments
Coeliac disease	Gluten-free diet	Exclude wheat, oats, rye, barley
Resistant coeliac disease	Soya-free Dairy product-free	Only some responsive
Crohn's disease	Elemental diet (or TPN)	Useful in acute phase of disease
Disaccharidase deficiency	Disaccharide-restricted diet	Lactase deficiency common (5% population) Sucrase-isomaltase deficiency rare
Small intestinal resection	High protein, low fat	Careful dietary manipulation to get optimal results
Irritable bowel	High fibre	Especially if associated with constipation
	Elimination diet	May help some especially with diarrhoea
Protein-losing enteropathy	Low fat High protein	Limits losses from blocked lymphatics May improve hepatic synthesis of albumin

Severe diarrhoea. Cholera, severe gastroenteritis, massive resection of the small intestine and neurohormonal disorders of gastrointestinal motility may cause life-threatening diarrhoea. The principles of management are straightforward. Fluid electrolytes and minerals must be replaced (intravenously if necessary) and the general nutritional state maintained. In the Tropics, apart from respiratory infection, acute diarrhoea is the most common cause of morbidity and mortality. In the early phase of acute infantile diarrhoea oral replacement of fluid (ORF) using a salt–sugar solution (Fig. 4.6) to make the best use of the mucosal pump has had a dramatic effect on survival.

Similar solutions are occasionally helpful in the management of patients with severe diarrhoea after a massive resection of small intestine.

Steatorrhoea. Steatorrhoea occurs in patients who have a disturbance in the complex mechanisms for fat absorption. It may be necessary to load the system (i.e. to give 100 g of fat a day) and to collect stools for at least 3 days in order to demonstrate steatorrhoea. Often the patient does not suffer diarrhoea. The common causes of steatorrhoea are:

1. Gastric surgery – Failure of mixing of food with pancreatic and biliary secretions.
2. Chronic pancreatitis – Loss of exocrine secretion.
3. Small intestinal pathology (especially coeliac disease and tropical sprue) – Digestive and absorptive failure.
4. Ileal dysfunction (especially Crohn's disease and intestinal resection) – Bile salt wasting and intestinal hurry.
5. Stagnant loop syndrome – Bacterial overgrowth; effect on micelle formation and mucosal function.

Patients with steatorrhoea frequently lose weight because they lose excess calories in their faeces and more significantly because they usually have reduced appetites. They also develop deficiencies of fat-soluble vitamins. The management of these patients depends on elucidating and correcting the cause of the malabsorption. If this is not possible it may be necessary to treat symptomatically with a low fat diet plus added vitamins. Long-chain fats in the diet may be replaced by medium-chain triglycerides but these are unpalatable and it is usually possible to provide sufficient energy by other means. Children with cystic fibrosis often have poor appetites and may benefit from intermittent tube feeding.

The large intestine

The principal function of the colon is to absorb water and electrolytes. It also provides a salvage pathway for unabsorbed carbohydrate and nitrogen. Bacterial metabolites from these substrates include volatile fatty acids and ammonia which are absorbed and enter body metabolic pathways. Fat is not used as an energy substrate by colonic bacteria; the fatty acids may be modified but are largely excreted in the faeces.

Fibre has an important effect on colonic function. It largely consists

Recognition and Management of Nutritional Disorders

TREATMENT OF GASTROENTERITIS – ORAL REPLACEMENT FLUID

Basic formula
Sodium chloride	3.5 g	(58 mmol)
Sodium bicarbonate	2.5 g	(30 mmol)
Potassium chloride	1.5 g	(20 mmol)
Glucose	20 g	(60 mmol)
Potable water	1 litre	

(Sucrose or rice starch may be substituted for glucose; 40 g sucrose gives a solution of equivalent osmolarity.)

Crude measure
A 3–4 finger scoop of sucrose	1 tablespoon	25 g (40 mmol)
Two pinches (thumb and two fingers) of salt	½ teaspoon	3 g (50 mmol)
Potable water	1 pint	574 ml

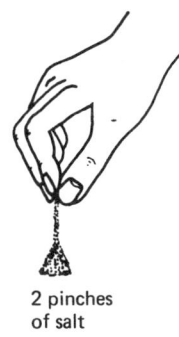

2 pinches of salt

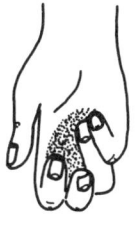

3–4 finger scoop of sugar

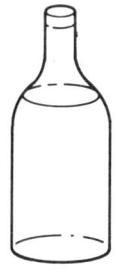

One pint of water

Figure 4.6 Oral replacement fluid. There are many variants on the basic formula which aims to produce a solution of approximately 280 mOsm/l to which sodium, and to a lesser extent potassium, salts contribute about two-thirds and the remainder comes from a simple carbohydrate (usually glucose or sucrose).

of cellulose, non-cellulosic polysaccharides and lignins. These are also partially metabolized by bacteria. The osmotic effect of the resulting small molecules and the increased bacterial mass makes the stools soft and bulky. Dietary fibre has important physiological effects (see Chapter 6, p. 180, Table 6.4).

It has been suggested that a high fibre diet protects against colonic disorders (see Table 6.2), coronary artery disease and gallstones, but direct evidence is lacking. For example, a high fibre diet produces only small changes in the concentration of circulating cholesterol and the epidemiological associations, especially with respect to atheroma, are not very convincing.

It is difficult to give firm guidelines on a desirable intake of fibre. The physiological effects of fibre vary with the dietary source. At present most authorities advise an intake of about 30 g a day. This is not easy to achieve. Four slices of white bread contain 3 g, whereas four slices of wholemeal bread contain 9 g. To achieve the recommended intake virtually all carbohydrate should be taken unrefined − bran cereal, potatoes, corn, beans, raw fruit and vegetables. Otherwise it is necessary deliberately to add bran to meals.

The advantages of a high fibre diet, apart from relief of constipation, may be considerably less than is often claimed. The disadvantages include increased flatulence; a possible increase in the incidence of colonic volvulus and intestinal intussusception; and, of uncertain significance, reduced absorption of divalent cations.

Liver disease

At present we do not know enough about the effect of diet on the physiological and biochemical disturbances which occur in hepato-biliary disease to give more than general guidelines on how diet may be used to minimize symptoms and improve prognosis.

In viral or drug hepatitis patients should be encouraged to eat normally. Dietary restrictions do not improve prognosis and there is some evidence to suggest that a high calorie intake may be beneficial. Fat does not need to be restricted and there is no evidence to show that alcohol in moderation has a deleterious effect. Nevertheless advice to abstain from alcohol can be justified in that relapses may be alcohol-related.

Gallstones are common and often associated with the nutritionally-related disorders of obesity, hypertriglyceridaemia and diabetes mellitus. In experimental animals, gallstones can be induced by a diet rich in refined carbohydrate and there is evidence to show that the addition of bran to a high carbohydrate diet makes bile less lithogenic. Nevertheless, many other factors are important in the pathogenesis of gallstones and dietary modification does not play a part in patient management. Often gallstones are discovered during the investigation of dyspepsia. Patients may relate their symptoms to the ingestion of fat although available evidence suggests that 'fatty food intolerance' is as common in patients without as in those with gallstones. It is logical, however, to limit fat intake in patients with obstructive biliary disease in order to reduce the secretion of cholecystokinin (CCK).

Patients with long-standing biliary obstruction (e.g. primary biliary cirrhosis) are unable to absorb fat normally. Hypoprothrombinaemia, secondary to vitamin K deficiency, occurs within a few weeks and must be treated with an appropriate parenteral preparation. Low grade deficiency of the other fat-soluble vitamins takes longer to develop. Synthesis of vitamin D may be impaired in jaundiced skin. The dietary component is therefore more important but may be poorly absorbed. As a result some patients with obstructive jaundice develop osteomalacia which frequently goes unrecognized unless it is actively considered using tests (serum calcium, phosphate and 25-hydroxycholecalciferol (25 HOCC); bone scanning and bone biopsy). Circulating alkaline phosphatase, which is usually the most sensitive marker of osteomalacia, will be helpful only if the biochemist can separate the increase due to bone disease from that caused by obstructive liver disease by the measurement of iso-enzymes.

Cirrhosis of the liver is a serious condition and dietary manipulation is often necessary in its management. In the well-compensated patient, dietary restriction (apart from the avoidance of alcohol) is usually unnecessary. Sometimes it may be necessary to limit the intake of carbohydrate because glucose tolerance is impaired and levels of circulating insulin are high as a result of the liver dysfunction. The incidence of insulin-dependent diabetes is also increased in patients with cirrhosis. Most patients with cirrhosis sooner or later develop fluid retention. A low salt diet (progressively reduced to 20 mmol/day) will help many patients clear the excess water. These patients must avoid salty foods, use unsalted bread and restrict their intake of protein to 60–70 g (because of the salt contained in protein foods). Diuretics are also given to such patients and some clinicians prefer to use drugs in preference to strict salt restriction.

A proportion of patients are unable to excrete free water. They become hyponatraemic yet remain oedematous. Fluid intake should be restricted to about 1 l/day. It is often best not to attempt to treat such patients too vigorously unless the retention of fluid is causing troublesome symptoms. The response to all forms of treatment is poor and life expectancy is short.

Hepatic encephalopathy is the most serious complication of liver disease. Dietary protein is an important aetiological factor but the exact mechanism of cerebral dysfunction remains uncertain. The principles of treatment are as follows:

1. Give no protein by mouth for 2–3 days.
2. Clear intestinal contents with purgatives.
3. Administer lactulose to minimize the absorption of ammonia.

Protein should be reintroduced gradually (by weekly increments of 10–20 g/day). The clinician aims to preserve nitrogen balance without allowing the redevelopment of encephalopathy. Protein from vegetables may be better tolerated than that from animal sources. Most patients can increase their intake to 40 g/day without serious symptoms.

Renal disease

Patients with renal failure frequently become malnourished. Attempts to maintain the intake of protein worsen symptoms and may accelerate the development of anaemia. Contrary to recent claims, the evidence that giving protein accelerates the deterioration of renal function is inconclusive. Nevertheless diet does have an important part to play in overall management.

Acute renal failure

Acute renal failure is usually the result of major trauma or of a severe disease process. Often the patient is unable to eat. He is resistant to insulin which reduces the intracellular availability of glucose and accelerates the mobilization of tissue protein. The period of recovery may take several weeks and a small proportion of patients will go on to develop chronic renal failure (see below). Current practice is to dialyse in order to maintain a good nutritional state. When dialysis is not possible, or before it is clear that it is needed, treatment should be ordered: to limit fluid intake to measured body losses (plus 500 ml for insensible evaporation), to meet caloric needs by giving at least 100 g glucose daily and to give sufficient amino acids to minimize the breakdown of body protein (equivalent to 3.5 g nitrogen). Few patients can tolerate such a highly restricted diet for more than a few days. This difficulty can be overcome by tube-feeding suitable liquid diets (e.g. Aminaid), although the high osmolality of such preparations may limit the volume which can be infused.

As methods of dialysis become easier acute renal failure is managed with more liberal dietary regimens – the frequency of dialysis being determined by renal function rather than by nutritional intake. Patients feel better when allowed to eat reasonably freely.

Many patients with acute renal failure are maintained on TPN. Essential amino acids 0.3–0.5 g/kg body weight should be given intravenously together with glucose and fat in high concentrations to limit the volume of fluid infused. Those on TPN maintain a better protein balance when given a mixture of essential and non-essential amino acids.

Chronic renal failure

The health of the patient with chronic renal failure not requiring dialysis is closely related to dietary intake. Protein intake is restricted in order to limit the accumulation of protein metabolites. With a creatinine clearance above 25 ml/min the patient may take 60–70 g protein/day. Below this level, protein intake should be progressively restricted down to 0.5–0.6 g/kg/day; 70% of the dietary protein should be of high biological value. If the creatinine clearance rate falls to around 5 ml/min or less it eventually becomes impossible to avoid uraemic symptoms and still maintain body protein status. A diet based on low-protein starch with supplements of non-starch carbohydrates provides the necessary calories. Sodium requirements will vary according to urine losses (50–150 mmol/day) potassium intake should be restricted to less than 70 mmol/day, although unless there is sudden deterioration in renal function, hyperkalaemia is usually not a problem.

Phosphate retention and hyperphosphataemia lead to hypocalcaemia and hyperparathyroidism. Calcium metabolism may also be disturbed by the inadequate conversion of 25 HOCC to 1:25 HOCC. The principles of treatment are as follows (in increasing order of magnitude):

1. ensure an adequate intake of vitamin D in all patients with renal failure (give vitamin supplement);
2. lower serum phosphate by giving aluminium hydroxide;
3. increase calcium intake by giving up to 20 g calcium gluconate orally;
4. control resistant hypocalcaemia with a 1α-hydroxylated preparation of vitamin D (or dihydrotachysterol);

5. treat osteomalacia with large doses of vitamin D.

Patients with chronic renal failure on restricted diets also need supplements of folic acid and water-soluble vitamins.

Maintenance dialysis. The factors causing malnutrition may be aggravated by maintenance dialysis. Up to 10 g of free amino acids are lost with each haemodialysis. Peptides, glucose, trace elements and water-soluble vitamins (especially folic acid, pyridoxine and ascorbic acid) are leached from the body. With peritoneal dialysis the losses are even greater, especially if the serosal membrane becomes inflamed. The principles of dietary treatment are as follows:

1. High intake of protein – 1.2 g/kg/day for haemodialysis and 1.7 g/kg/day for peritoneal dialysis.
2. High normal calorie intake – 35 kcal (145 kJ)/kg/day. (Hyperlipidaemia is common so encourage intake of complex carbohydrates and polyunsaturated fatty acids.)
3. Intake of sodium tailored to requirements according to limits of renal ability to conserve and secrete sodium ions (usually 40–100 mmol/day).
4. Intake of potassium limited to 40–70 mmol according to situation.
5. Supplements of trace elements – Iron = ferrous sulphate 300 mg t.d.s. and zinc = zinc sulphate 200 mg daily.
6. Supplements of water-soluble vitamins – folic acid = 1 mg per day; pyridoxine = 10 mg per day; ascorbic acid = 100 mg per day. Vitamin B12 is not required and vitamin A should not be given routinely because circulating levels rise in uraemic patients.

Food allergy and food intolerance

Abnormal reactions to foods and food additives undoubtedly occur in some subjects (Table 4.18) but extravagant therapeutic claims without sound clinical or scientific evidence have produced a confused picture.

Food intolerance may occur because of:

1. Associated toxins – Contaminated foodstuffs (e.g. cooking oil adulterated with tricresyl phosphate).

Table 4.18 *Some food-related acquired diseases*

Proven
  Coeliac disease
  Cows' milk protein intolerance
  Dermatitis herpetiformis
Possible in some cases
  Urticaria, angio-oedema
  Migraine
  Atopic eczema
  Cot death
  Asthma, rhinitis, conjunctivitis
  Irritable bowel syndrome
Unproven
  Inflammatory bowel disease
  Rheumatoid arthritis
  Multiple sclerosis
  Hyperkinetic behaviour in children

Note: The so-called 'total allergy syndrome' is a psychiatric disorder.

2. Direct pharmacological action – e.g. Tyramine in cheese, caffeine in beverages.
3. Indirect pharmacological action – e.g. Release of histamine by tomatoes or strawberries.
4. Local irritant action – Spicy foods.
5. Failure of a digestive process – e.g. Lactose in lactase deficient subjects.
6. Failure of intermediary metabolism – e.g. Protein intolerance in phenylketonuria.
7. IgE mediated hypersensitivity – e.g. Urticaria due to fish.
8. Defined sensitivity (with objective response to challenge – gluten sensitivity, cows milk protein intolerance).
9. Apparent sensitivity (usually only subjective response to challenge) – Asthma, irritable bowel syndrome.

There is little difficulty in advising the patient who describes a clear cut relationship between a foodstuff and disease, e.g. cheese or chocolate-induced headaches, strawberry-induced urticaria or milk-induced diarrhoea. Similarly the recognition of a pathological process known to be caused by diet presents no problems; coeliac disease and dermatitis herpetiformis are good examples.

The problem is knowing how best to help the patient who might have food intolerance when there is no clear cut relationship of symptoms to food ingestion and no objective means of measuring the response. Available tests are largely unsatisfactory (Table 4.19). It is part of

Table 4.19 Diagnostic tests for food allergy and intolerance

Test	Comment
Prick tests	Limited value Positive tests may persist long after allergic response has disappeared Well-defined immediate skin reactions (>5 mm) and positive RAST to the same allergens may help define IgE hypersensitivity Delayed reactions of no clinical value
Radioallergosorbent test (RAST)	Detects specific IgE antibody to foods (but must be interpreted with care)
IgG antibodies to food	Poor correlation with disease Positive in coeliac disease, inflammatory bowel disease (probably reflects increased intestinal permeability)
Provocation tests	Very difficult to perform objectively At present the only method of testing for food allergy
Hair analysis Sublingual provocation tests Pulse tests Cytotoxic tests Intradermal injection	Validity of all these tests is extremely dubious

human behaviour to seek a cause for observed effects and it is easy to convince oneself that the attack of abdominal pain was due to egg taken for breakfast – an hour ago, a day ago, or even a week ago. But when, on an egg-free diet the pain recurs the hunt for a possible cause may reach ridiculous proportions. Was that mayonnaise really free of egg? Or is another food responsible?

Clinicians with an interest in nutrition will have their patience and skill tested to the ultimate by subjects who believe their symptoms of weakness, lethargy, blackouts, chest pain, difficulty in breathing, palpitations, headaches, disorders of bowel or bladder habit, abdominal pain, aching joints and parasthesiae are due to food intolerance. The symptoms are often diffuse, always non-specific and usually not associated with physical signs except those which can be produced at will (e.g. hyperventilation).

The following sequence of investigation is suggested:

1. Take a careful clinical history.
2. Look hard for evidence of organic disease.
3. Take a full dietary history.
4. Assess organ function where indicated – e.g. Simple lung studies in patients with wheezing, exercise tolerance in patients with weakness, tests of intestinal permeability in patients with diarrhoea.
5. Repeat the clinical history noting – Degree of concordance with previous history, possible psychosocial factors influencing disease, apparent precipitating factors for disease.
6. Decide whether or not to investigate diet further.
7. If food intolerance appears to be a likely cause of disease then trial of an elimination diet.

A full dietary history by a skilled dietition may indicate possible causes of intolerance. For example the patient who drinks 20 cups of tea a day may be suffering from the effect of caffeine and tannin, excess fibre intake may cause excessive flatulence and diarrhoea.

If the clinician decides to recommend a trial of food elimination he would be wise to ensure that the patient is sensible enough to follow the programme, is well-motivated and is free of obvious neuroses. Food intolerance may be assessed quite simply by prescribing a diet free of foods which are most commonly claimed as offenders (wheat, dairy products, eggs, chocolate, fish, nuts, tomatoes and strawberries). If symptoms are improved on a restricted diet, new foods may be introduced one at a time to try to identify an offending agent. A small proportion of patients with symptoms of irritable bowel or migraine undoubtedly respond well. The symptoms of patients presenting with non-specific abdominal pain and intermittent diarrhoea are particularly interesting because they appear to offer the best chance of determining mechanisms of food intolerance.

A more rigorous programme starts with a diet consisting solely of lamb pears and spring water. It is difficult to manage and is used mainly by clinicians with a special interest in food intolerance. Patients must be selected with care. The neurotically anxious will find plenty of scope to indulge their phobias and fantasies and the clinician may find that his clinical practice is flooded by patients described in a *Lancet* editorial as 'pseudo-allergic'.

FURTHER READING

Protein-calorie malnutrition

Coward W. A., Lunn P. (1981). The biochemistry and physiology of kwashiorkor and marasmus. *Brit. Med. Bull*; 37: 19–24.

Williams C. D. (1933). A nutritional disease of childhood associated with a maize diet. *Arch. Dis. Childh*; 8: 423–33.

World Health Organization. (1981). *The Treatment and Management of Severe Protein-calorie Malnutrition*. Geneva: WHO.

Anorexia

Crisp A. H. (1980). *Anorexia Nervosa*. London: Academic Press.

Anaemia

Lindenbaum J., ed. (1983). *Nutrition in Haematology*. Edinburgh: Churchill Livingstone.

Osteopenic bone disease

DHSS. (1980). Report on Health and Social Subjects, No. 19. *Rickets and Osteomalacia*. London: HMSO.

Heath D., Marx S. J., eds. (1982). *Calcium Disorders*. London: Butterworths.

NIH Consensus Conference. (1984). Treatment and prevention of osteoporosis. *JAMA*; **252**: 799–802.

Obesity

Garrow J. S. (1981). *Treat Obesity Seriously*. Edinburgh: Churchill Livingstone.

NIH Consensus Conference. (1985). Health implications of obesity. *Int. J. Obesity*; 9: 155–70.

Stunkard A. J. (1980). *Obesity*. Philadelphia: W. B. Saunders Co.

Stunkard A. J., Stellar E., eds. (1984). *Eating and its Disorders*. (Association for Research in Nervous and Mental Disease. Research publication series: Vol. 62.) New York: Raven Press.

Stunkard A. J., Sørensen T. I., Hanis C., *et al.* (1986). An adoption study of human obesity. *New Engl. J. Med*; **314**: 193–8.

Hyperlipidaemia

Lewis B. (1976). *The Hyperlipidaemias. Clinical and Laboratory Practice.* Oxford: Blackwell Scientific Publications.
NIH Consensus Conference (1983). Treatment of hypertriglyceridaemia. *JAMA*; **251**: 1196–200.
NIH Consensus Conference. (1985). Lowering blood cholesterol. *JAMA*; **253**: 2080–6.

Nutrition and alcohol

Spring J., Buss D. H. (1977). Three centuries of alcohol in the British diet. *Nature*; **270**: 567–72.

Nutrition and drugs

Buchanan N. (1984). Effect of malnutrition on drug metabolism in man. *World Rev. Nutr. Diet*; **43**: 129–39.

Diabetes

Oakley W. G., Pyke D. A., Taylor K. G. (1980). *Diabetes and its Management.* Oxford: Blackwell Scientific Publications.
Simpson H. C. R., Simpson R. W., Lonsley S., *et al.* (1981). A high carbohydrate leguminous fibre diet improves all aspects of diabetic control. *Lancet*; **1**: 1–5.

Nutrition and gastrointestinal disorders

Heatley V., Kelleher J., Losowsky M. (1986). Clinical nutrition. In *Gastroenterology.* Edinburgh: Churchill Livingstone.

Food allergy and food intolerance

Hunter J. O., Alun Jones V., eds. (1985). *Food and the Gut.* London: Baillière Tindall.
NIH Consensus Conference. (1982). Defined diets and childhood hyperactivity. *JAMA*; **248**: 290–3.

Chapter 5

Nutritional Support

ENCOURAGING THE PATIENT TO EAT • MAKING BEST USE OF THE GUT – PHYSIOLOGICAL PRINCIPLES • THE FORMULATION OF DIETS FOR ARTIFICIAL ENTERAL FEEDING • ENTERAL DIETS • TUBE FEEDING • ADMINISTRATION OF FEEDS • TOTAL PARENTERAL NUTRITION (TPN) • MEETING REQUIREMENTS BY THE INTRAVENOUS ROUTE • DELIVERY SYSTEMS • COMPLICATIONS OF TPN • HOME PARENTERAL NUTRITION • THE NUTRITION TEAM • FURTHER READING

Interest in systems of nutritional support has been stimulated by reports that most patients admitted to hospital with serious illness leave less well-nourished than when admitted. Indeed it has been suggested that hospitals are the major reservoir of malnutrition in the UK. Moreover there are many reports suggesting that undernutrition is an important cause of morbidity and mortality after major surgery. Whether this is so or not is debatable, but certainly there is no reason for such patients to be semistarved for long periods.

The basic rules for nutritional support are straightforward:

1. Assess the patient's nutritional state.
2. Correct specific deficiencies by the most appropriate means.
3. Observe and record the dietary intake.
4. When necessary supplement dietary intake by the simplest available route.

Practice often falls short of precept. In particular, it is difficult to get an accurate impression of how well the patient has been eating, particularly as nurses no longer routinely supervise meals.

ENCOURAGING THE PATIENT TO EAT

Often too little time is spent tempting the sick person to eat. This is particularly true for the elderly. It is important to be aware of factors

Nutritional Support

associated with long-standing poor food intake (Table 5.1) as well as the effects of acute disease. The clinician who shows an interest will usually get a positive response from nurses, dietitians and relatives. It is their care, attention and cooperation which may be vital in improving the ability of the sick patient to maintain his nutritional state by physiological means. Patients with dysphagia need special encouragement. Often they can keep eating by avoiding those foods that stick and by liquidizing their main meals. Some patients find it difficult to eat a sufficient amount of food particularly if they are sick and underweight. Such patients need nutritional support which should be provided by the simplest possible means (Table 5.2).

MAKING BEST USE OF THE GUT – PHYSIOLOGICAL PRINCIPLES

In providing nutritional support the clinician must be able to assess how best to use the gastrointestinal tract. This requires some knowledge of factors affecting the normal physiology of digestion and absorption (Table 5.3).

Delivery of food to the small intestine

Food is swallowed as a masticated bolus mixed with salivary amylase and pharyngeal lipase. In the stomach it is converted to a liquid chyme in the presence of acid and pepsin. Intrinsic factor is added for the absorption of vitamin B12. The chyme is metered into the duodenum where it meets bile and pancreatic secretions. These produce the molecular structures which can be handled by the digestive–absorptive surface of the small intestine – the brush border of the enterocyte.

Carbohydrate

Carbohydrate must be reduced to monosaccharides (mol. wt. 180) before absorption. Unless these are taken up quickly they will have a major osmotic effect in the lumen of the intestine. Thus the arrival of carbohydrate in the small intestine is believed to be the key factor in the syndrome of early dumping. This occurs particularly in patients who have a gastroenterostomy and it may also be a problem with the infusion of a hyperosmolar solution of nutrients directly into the small

Table 5.1 *Factors associated with prolonged poor food intake in the elderly who do not have serious pathology*

Medical
    Poorly fitting dentures
    Difficulty in swallowing
    Previous gastric surgery
Social
    Housebound
    Social classes IV and V
    In receipt of Supplementary Benefit
    No regular cooked meals

From: DHSS. (1979). Report on Health and Social Subjects, No. 16. *Nutrition and Health in Old Age.* London: HMSO.

Table 5.2 *Methods of nutritional support*

Route	Means
Oral	Dietary supplements
	Artificial enteral feeds
Nasoenteral	Liquid enteral feed
Direct enteral	Liquid enteral feed
Peripheral venous	Dextrose, lipid, electrolyte and isotonic amino acid solutions
Central venous	Hypertonic TPN solutions

intestine. The carbohydrate energy content of enteral diets may be increased without disturbing osmolarity by substituting high molecular weight glucose polymers for mono- and disaccharides. Such carbohydrates (e.g. Caloreen and Hycal) are useful supplements in enteral feeding.

The brush border disaccharidases are important for the digestion and uptake of glucose polymers (both artificial and those produced by the digestion of starch), lactose and sucrose. Adult brush border lactase deficiency is a common condition (5% of the British indiginous population, 20% of non-Caucasian Europeans and near to 100% of non-milk drinking Afro–Asian ethnic groups). This is an important consideration as artificial enteric feeds are usually milk-based. Nevertheless most subjects can take small quantities (25–50 g lactose)

Table 5.3 Intestinal capacity

Nutrient	Absorptive capacity	Comments
Carbohydrate	Big reserve	Colon absorbs 2–6%
Protein	Small intestine >90%	(after fermentation)
Fat	To more than 350 g	No colonic absorption (Diet 50–350 g Faeces 4–10 g)
Fat-soluble vitamins	50–90% intake	Vitamin K from bacteria
Water-soluble vitamins	Mega-doses absorbed easily	Malabsorption rarely a problem
Vitamin B12	1–2 µg only	Limited by ileal transport
Calcium	30–60% of intake (75% in children)	Influenced by previous dietary intake and D status
Magnesium	50% of intake	Control not well understood (Vitamin D has limited effect)
Iron	Very variable Diet (Up to 60% haem iron) (Up to 10% non-haem iron)	Controlled by gut mucosa especially duodenum Enhanced by: gastric acid, ferric salt, >ferrous vitamin C
	Absorption of iron salts	
		Normal / Iron deficient
	0.5 mg dose	25% / 75%
	50 mg dose	5% / 20%

without serious side-effects. Isomaltase-sucrase deficiency is extremely rare and usually there is a history of diarrhoea from childhood.

Protein

Protein is well absorbed from the gastrointestinal tract. The secretion of pepsin is not a limiting step for protein digestion, although it may become so in subjects with pancreatic insufficiency (certainly a patient with a partial gastrectomy who develops pancreatic insufficiency will have life-threatening malabsorption). The exocrine function of the pancreas has considerable reserve capacity (perhaps 10-fold), and thus most patients needing nutritional support can be fed a diet containing whole protein as the source of nitrogen.

The breakdown products of protein are absorbed primarily as short-chain peptides. These have a kinetic advantage over amino acids in crossing the brush border of the small intestine. Thus in the patient with a very short small intestine (in whom there appears to be inadequate time for digestion), and in the patient in whom the clinician suspects protein intolerance, it may be reasonable to give a liquid feed containing oligopeptides as the source of nitrogen. There seems to be little place for elemental diets in which nitrogen is in the form of free amino acids. Oligopeptide-containing diets are cheaper and carry a lower osmotic load than elemental diets. Regrettably they are only marginally more palatable and relatively few patients can tolerate these liquid feeds by mouth for prolonged periods (see Table 5.5).

Lipids

The major dietary lipids comprise triglycerides, cholesterol and the fat-soluble vitamins A, D, E and K. Absorptive processes require pancreatic lipase, bile acids, a well-functioning small intestine and an adequate lymphatic drainage. The body's reserve for fat absorption is considerable, but steatorrhoea is a common manifestation of malabsorption because fat is not used as an energy substrate by intestinal bacteria.

Triglycerides are an important source of energy but carbohydrate may act as a substitute. Low fat enteral feeds are indicated in patients with cholestatic jaundice, severe pancreatic insufficiency, massive resection of the small intestine or severe mucosal disorders (e.g. gluten-insensitive enteropathy, radiation enteritis) and intestinal lymph-angiectasia. Medium-chain triglycerides (MCT) are sometimes substituted for long-chain triglycerides in enteral feeds. There is some evidence that MCT may be hydrolyzed by pharyngeal lipase and that MCT may be absorbed without micellar solubilization. Thus MCT provides a possible means for increasing energy intake from enteral feeds. In practice the advantages appear marginal and MCT is rarely needed for the maintenance of patients with severe malabsorption. Cholesterol is not a critical dietary nutrient. It is, of course, a vital component of cell membranes for which the body has adequate synthetic mechanisms. Deficiency of fat-soluble vitamins is common in patients with long-standing malabsorption. Artificial diets often contain more than the recommended dietary allowances but absorption may be impaired sufficiently seriously to make parenteral supplementation necessary.

Water-soluble vitamins

Apart from folic acid and vitamin B12, a deficiency of water-soluble vitamins is rare in gastrointestinal disease. Folic acid deficiency is common in malnourished subjects. This is usually due to a combination of poor dietary intake and increased requirements rather than poor digestion and absorption. The increased requirements for folic acid in inflammatory and neoplastic disorders have not been well defined. Patients with severe mucosal enteropathy in the jejunum (coeliac disease, tropical sprue) are unable to absorb sufficient folic acid from normal dietary folate. In such cases the requirements of about 100 µg/day may be met by an oral supplement (Tab. Folic Acid 5 mg/day).

Vitamin B12 deficiency occurs much less commonly. Stores in the normal liver will cover body needs for 3–5 years. Nevertheless after total gastrectomy or ileal resection it will be necessary to provide Vitamin B12 by intramuscular injection (hydroxycobalamin 1000 µg every 3 months).

Minerals

The absorptive processes for minerals are fundamentally different from those of carbohydrate, protein and fat. They provide important control mechanisms for body homeostasis. Thus body iron status is regulated by absorption from the gut and to some extent this holds true for calcium and possibly magnesium. Calcium excretion is controlled by the kidney but this has a physiological limit (persistent hypercalcuria leads to the precipitation of calcium salts in the urine). The percentage of calcium absorbed by the gut reduces with increasing intake. This provides the body with an additional protective mechanism.

Iron

Iron deficiency is common in patients requiring nutritional support. The average diet has little reserve to cover a failing appetite or low grade malabsorption. Iron is best absorbed from the duodenum. Thus iron deficiency is nearly universal in patients with a long-standing gastroenterostomy. Absorption from enteral feeds is very variable. In the ordinary diet up to 60% of haem iron (i.e. from meat) may be absorbed but less than 10% of non-haem iron. Absorption of iron from inorganic salts depends on the dose and iron status of the patient as well as on absorptive function. In a healthy person with a normal small intestine, 25% of a 0.5 mg dose will be absorbed but only 5% of a 50 mg dose. With iron deficiency these figures increase 3-fold. Most artificial enteral diets contain inorganic iron salts. It may be necessary to supplement these feeds particularly in the patient with a diseased or bypassed duodenum. It is important to check the patient's iron status from time to time because the majority of patients requiring artificial nutrition are anaemic. Often, however, the anaemia is not due to iron deficiency. In such circumstances it is wrong to give large quantities of iron thereby over-riding the body's defence mechanisms.

Calcium

The absorption of calcium is controlled by a complex set of mechanisms involving vitamin D, parathormone, cortisol and possibly other pituitary controlled hormones. There is an adaptation to dietary intake, and absorption falls with age and some disorders, e.g. renal insufficiency. Calcium cannot be absorbed if it is precipitated as an insoluble salt or complex. Phytate present in low extraction flour diminishes calcium absorption although in acute studies adaptation has been shown to occur after a few weeks.

Calcium is absorbed chiefly in the jejunum where the rather low pH (6.0) favours the solubilization of calcium salts more than the more alkaline contents of the ileum. In practice when patients are given artificial enteral feeds their intake of calcium is usually markedly increased because such feeds are milk-based. It is important, however, to maintain the vitamin D status, especially in patients who have little or no access to sunlight.

Magnesium

The absorption of magnesium is slower than that of calcium and the cellular mechanism is incompletely understood. Vitamin D appears to increase absorption but the importance of this finding is not known. Magnesium deficiency is not uncommon in clinical practice, especially in alcoholics and in patients with serious pathology of the small intestine. It is not always easy to correct magnesium deficiency by giving magnesium salts orally because they may cause diarrhoea (see Table 3.11).

Phosphorus

Dietary phosphates are well absorbed and unlike the divalent cations the intestine exerts relatively little control. Body content is regulated by urinary excretion which under normal conditions is equivalent to about 70% of intake. Ordinary food and artificial complete feeds contain enough phosphorus for normal requirements but hypophosphataemia occurs quite commonly during the nutritional repletion of malnourished subjects (see Table 3.10).

Zinc and copper

Relatively little is known about the absorption of zinc and copper from artificial feeds. Unfortunately there is at present no simple method of assessing marginal nutritional status with respect to these two trace elements. Care must be taken if supplements are given over a prolonged period. Magnesium and zinc will reduce the absorption of iron; conversely, iron interferes with the absorption of zinc. These interactions are probably significant only with pharmacological doses.

Water and electrolytes

The handling of water and electrolytes by the intestine is often the limiting factor in artificial enteral nutrition. Under normal circumstances the adult gut absorbs nearly 10 l of fluid a day (6 ml/min) (Table 5.4). In the jejunum water and salt absorption are closely related to the

Table 5.4 Normal fluxes

	Input			Absorption			Excretion
	Diet	Secretions	Total	Small intestine	Large intestine	Total	Faecal
Water (l)	1.5	7.5	9.0	7.4 (17.0)*	1.5 (3.0)*	8.9 (20.0)*	0.1
Sodium (mmol)	150	1000	1150	950 (2500)*	195 (500)*	1145 (3000)*	5
Potassium (mmol)	80	40	120	110	−2	108	12
Chloride (mmol)	150	750	900	800	97	897	3

*Figures in brackets give an estimate of total absorptive capacity.

absorption of protein and carbohydrate. In the ileum and colon absorption is largely independent of nutrients. Sodium is actively absorbed and water follows passively. The transfer of chloride is to some extent independent of sodium and occurs at a faster rate against a steeper gradient. Bicarbonate is exchanged for chloride.

Under normal circumstances the contents of the duodenum are nearly isotonic. If hypertonic solutions are infused, water and electrolytes flood into the lumen of the bowel and may exceed its capacity for absorption. This has practical importance. Enteral feeds should be nearly isotonic and given slowly by controlled continuous infusion.

THE FORMULATION OF DIETS FOR ARTIFICIAL ENTERAL FEEDING

Consideration of the physiological principles outlined above indicate how to formulate enteral feeds.

Patients with an intact gastrointestinal tract

For the patient with a normal gut it would be best to give a homogenized normal diet. In practice this is often inconvenient and one of the many commercial preparations may be used. This should contain adequate amounts of first class protein for the patient's needs and calories according to perceived requirements. Most liquid diets contain approximately 1 kcal (4.2 kJ) per ml of formulation. The proportion of fat to carbohydrate is rarely of much importance, but the osmolality of the feed should be close to 285–300 mOsm/kg. The diet should contain adequate electrolytes, minerals, trace elements and vitamins.

Dietary adjustment for patients with impaired gastrointestinal function

In the patient with a gastrointestinal disorder, the clinician must delineate the defect as far as possible and adjust the enteral feed accordingly.

Carbohydrate absorption may be improved by using a solution containing glucose polymers and avoiding lactose. Nitrogen needs are sometimes best met by using a predigested diet containing oligopeptides rather than free amino acids. In patients with steatorrhoea the

Nutritional Support

fat content of the diet should be limited although enough given to satisfy the requirements for essential fatty acids (for an adult equivalent to about 10 g linoleic acid/day or 3% of the dietary energy). Some fat is also desirable because it provides abundant energy with little effect on osmolarity.

ENTERAL DIETS

Available preparations

There are several palatable high protein, energy dense liquid feeds which may be used to boost the normal dietary intake of the undernourished. Such feeds should be offered between meals and every effort must be made to satisfy the individual palate. Sick people have fickle appetites. That which is acceptable one day may be deemed unappetizing the next, so it is as well to have several feeds to hand. Many patients prefer milk-based liquid feeds to be served chilled. The amount offered should be within the patient's capacity and half empty drinks should not be left lying on the bedside locker. Unfortunately, many patients are rapidly sated by oral liquid feeds and it is then necessary to decide whether or not to tube-feed.

Tube-feeding provides the means of giving liquid nutrients directly into the gastrointestinal tract. Usually this is via the nasogastric route but in some cases it may be better to position the tube in the small intestine either via the nares or via a gastrostomy or an enterostomy. Patients are best fed by continuous infusion over 24 h. Many preparations are available and the dietician can advise the clinician which preparation is best able to satisfy the physiological needs (Table 5.5).

Hospital enteral feeds

It is possible for hospitals to produce their own tube feeds but in practice this is not cost-effective. The preparation of feeds is time-consuming, it is difficult to get the osmolality right and impossible to ensure that such feeds remain bacteriologically clean. Several centres have reported outbreaks of gastroenteritis related to hospital-prepared feeds. Even the large manufacturers may run in to trouble. The makers of Complan, which was a usual constituent of hospital feeds as well as a popular commercial food supplement, went out of business as a result of bacterial contamination of one of their baby feeds.

Table 5.5 *Liquid enteral feeds*

Approximate contents of standard full-strength feeds (per litre)
   1000 kcals (4.2 MJ) (approx)
   27–36 g protein (4.5–6.0 g nitrogen)
   33–42 g fat
   Appropriate vitamins and minerals
Oral Feeds
   Reasonably well tolerated oral feeds (omolarity 430–570)
     Build-up (Carnation)—60 g protein if made up with milk
     Ensure* (Abbott)
     Fortisip* (Cow and Gate)
Tube Feeds (with satisfactory flow through fine-bore tubes
   Whole protein tube feeds (osmolarity 350–400):

Clinifeed 400	(Roussel)
Clinifeed Favour*	(Roussel)
Fortison	(Cow and Gate)
Isocal*	(Mead Johnson)
Nutrauxil(*)	(Kabi–Vitrum)

   High energy tube feeds

Ensure Plus*	(Abbott)
Fortison Energy Plus	(Cow and Gate)
Two Cal HN*	(Abbott)

   High protein tube feeds (60–80 g/l)

Ensure (made up with milk)	(Abbott)
Clinifeed Protein Rich	(Roussel)
Two Cal HN*	(Abbott)

Feeds isosmolar with intestinal contents

Clinifeed Iso	(Roussel)
Fortisip*	(Cow and Gate)
Osmolite*	(Abbott)

* = Lactose-free.
(*) = Lactose-trace.
Note: Fortison range of feeds also includes a low sodium, a low protein/low mineral, and a soya-based feed.

Ideally home-made artificial enteral feeds should be pasteurized before being given to patients but for most hospitals this would be hopelessly impractical.

Proprietary enteral feeds

Some of the more popular proprietary enteral feeds are listed in Table 5.5. Whole protein feeds are suitable for most patients. They are all low

Nutritional Support

residue and most are satisfactory for the majority of patients. In some cases it may be wise to prescribe feeds which are lactose-free, low fat – high MCT, or of low osmolality (Table 5.6).

It is difficult to give clearcut advice regarding the desirable intake of protein and of calories. Most patients seem to do reasonably well on about 12 g nitrogen (75 g protein)/day and 1500–2000 kcal (6.3–8.4 MJ). Occasionally it may be helpful to estimate nitrogen requirements by measuring nitrogen loss (see Chapter 3, p. 54). This may be calculated crudely but sufficiently accurately for clinical purposes by the formula:

Nitrogen loss (g/24 h) = 2 + Urinary urea (mmol/day) ($\times$ 0.028 $\times$ 1.2)

The formula must be modified if the blood urea is changing in a consistent fashion or if the patient has abnormal nitrogen losses from the kidney or gut (see p. 54). (Note that most patients with protein-losing enteropathy do not have high levels of faecal nitrogen. They resorb the leaked nitrogen as amino acids much of which appears in the urine as urea. Excess nitrogen losses from the gut occur most often in patients with gastrointestinal fistulae.)

It is not possible to maintain a positive nitrogen balance for prolonged periods unless the patient has lost a lot of weight and is capable of taking a reasonable amount of exercise. Increasing the nitrogen intake of immobilized patients will often do no more than increase the metabolic load on the liver and kidneys.

It is possible to modulate the weight of patients by manipulating the caloric intake. Sometimes a prolonged illness will help an obese patient to lose weight and this opportunity should not be lost by an over-zealous provision of calories. The patient's weight should be monitored. The principle objective is to maintain active tissue mass. This can be assessed crudely by standard liver function tests and by measuring muscle mass and strength. It is important to remember that protein synthesis requires energy, principally from carbohydrate. Thus it is not sufficient to give protein alone.

TUBE FEEDING

Ryle's tube

Up until 1975 liquid feeds were given in boluses via a medium or wide bore nasogastric tube (Ryle's tube). This method is uncomfortable for

Table 5.6 *Liquid enteral feeds* (modified for intestinal disorders)

Whole protein feeds with a low content of LCT (high MCT)
    Osmolite   (Abbot)   19 g MCT   19 g LCT per litre
    Portagen   (Mead Johnson)   27 g MCT   7 g LCT
    Triosorbon   (Merck)   32 g MCT   8 g LCT

Non-milk whole protein feeds
    Fortison Soya   (Cow and Gate)   Soya protein
    Prosobee   (Mead Johnson)   Soya protein

Oligopeptide feeds (variable osmolarity)
    Flexical   (Mead Johnson)   Hydrolysed casein
    Nutramigen   (Mead Johnson)   Hydrolysed casein
    Peptide 2+   (SHS)   Hydrolysed meat and soya
    Reabilan   (Roussel)   Hydrolysed whey/casein

Oligopeptide feeds (low in LCT—high MCT)
    MCT Peptide   (SHS)   31 g MCT   6 g LCT per litre
    Nutranel   (Roussel)   5 g MCT   5 g LCT
    Peptisorbon   (Merck)   9 g MCT   6 g LCT
    Pregestimil   (Mead Johnson)   11 g MCT   16 g LCT

Amino Acid feeds (high osmolarity, low in fat)
    Elemental 028   (Scientific Hospital Supplies)
    Vivonex   (Norwich-Eaton)

Note Feeds suitable for infants (low sodium content)
    Portagen   (Mead Johnson)   Caseinate, low LCT, high MCT
    Prosobee   (Mead Johnson)   Soy protein
    Nutramigen   (Mead Johnson)   Hydrolysed casein
    Peptide 0–2   (SHS)   Hydrolysed meat and soya
    MCT Peptide 0–2 (SHS)   Hydrolysed meat and soya
                                                                   23 g MCT 5 g LCT
    Pregestimil   (Mead Johnson)   Hydrolysed casein
                                                                   11 g MCT 16 g LCT

the patient, is likely to cause dumping and diarrhoea, and may cause oesophageal ulceration. A Ryle's tube remains useful for feeding the patient with disturbed gastric function. If the tip is correctly placed, the stomach can be emptied every hour or so and this provides a useful safeguard against regurgitation of contents and subsequent aspiration pneumonia. Such tubes should not be used for routine feeding for periods of more than a few days. If the stomach empties poorly and recovery is likely to be delayed then it is better to pass a tube into the small intestine. In the short-term, drugs, such as metoclopramide, may be used to encourage gastric emptying but prolonged administration is

Nutritional Support

undesirable, especially in the elderly, because of potential side-effects on the central nervous system.

Simple fine-bore tubes

Fine-bore tubes have become popular for enteral feeding. They are passed into the stomach with the aid of an introducer (Fig. 5.1) and for most patients a simple unweighted, open-ended feeding tube works well. The clinician must ensure that:

1. The tube is correctly positioned.
2. The tube is not regurgitated when the patient coughs or retches.
3. The stomach empties satisfactorily.

It is also necessary to remember that although slow infusion of nutrients is an excellent method of feeding, the patient is deprived of the social contact which accompanies normal meals. It is possible to drink with a fine tube in position and when possible this should be encouraged.

Weighted tubes

A mercury-tipped tube is useful for intubating the patient with partial oesophageal obstruction (e.g. when there is an endotracheal tube in place) and for feeding directly into the duodenum or first part of the jejunum. Direct infusion into the small intestine reduces the risk of aspiration pneumonia. This is an important consideration in patients with disorders of the pharynx, with free gastro-oesophageal reflux and with gastric atony or obstruction.

Endoscopic placement of tubes

Some patients find it impossible to swallow a nasogastric tube. This is particularly true if there is organic narrowing or neuromuscular dysfunction of the oesophagus. In such patients endoscopic placement of the tube may be necessary (Fig. 5.2).

Percutaneous tube feeding

Some surgeons practice early postoperative feeding via a fine needle-catheter jejunostomy. This is not necessary for most patients under-

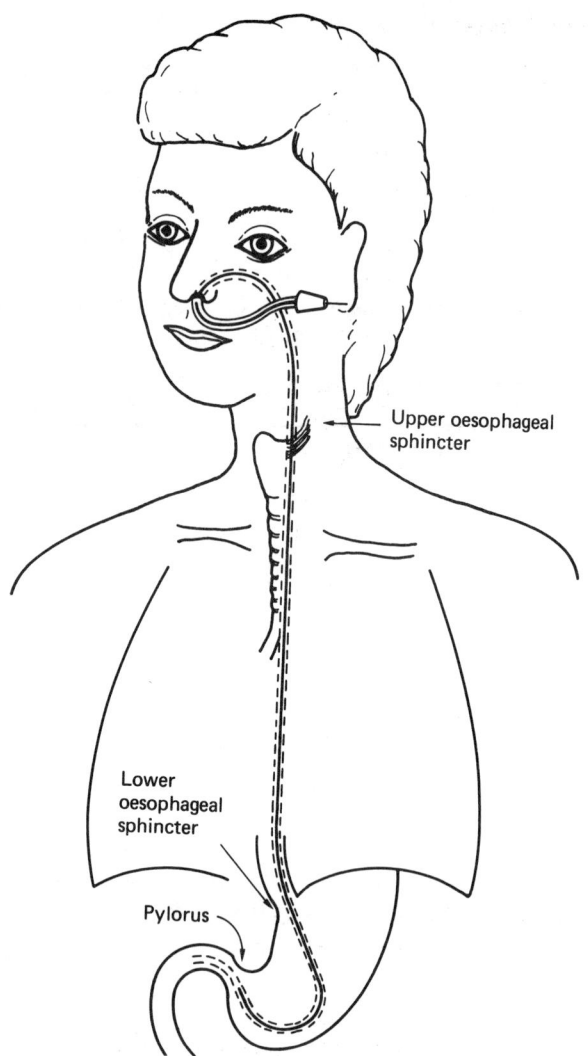

Figure 5.1 Fine-bore enteral feeding tube. The tube is stiffened by a central wire which cannot protrude from the tip. Normally the tube comes to rest in the body of the stomach or in the antrum. Regurgitation is prevented by the competence of the lower oesophageal sphincter. The upper oesophageal sphincter is not a sufficient barrier against reflux into the pharynx, but the trachea is normally protected by the cough reflex. If gastric emptying is delayed or if there is free reflux it may be necessary to use a long tube and to pass it through the pylorus into the small intestine under radiological control.

Nutritional Support

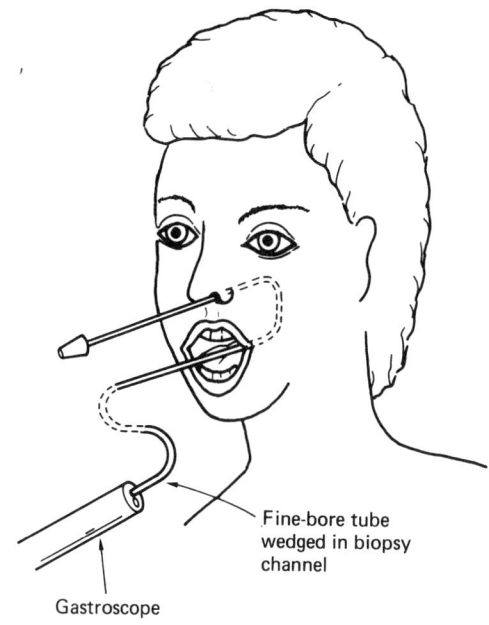

Figure 5.2 Methods of placing an enteral tube using a gastroduodendoscope.

going gastrointestinal surgery although it may be helpful in the occasional case of oesophagogastric obstruction. Long-term feeding via gastrostomy or enterostomy (Fig. 5.3) is sometimes indicated in patients with severe neurological disorders.

ADMINISTRATION OF FEEDS

Liquid enteral feeds are best given from a reservoir via an appropriate giving set. These are now designed so that they cannot be attached to an intravenous cannula. Liquid feeds in sealed cans or bottles are sterile and they can be poured into 2 l containers without significant bacterial contamination. It is then possible to infuse the contents of the reservoir over 24 h. Powdered preparations have to be made up with water. The use of a blender adds to the risk of contaminating a powdered feed.

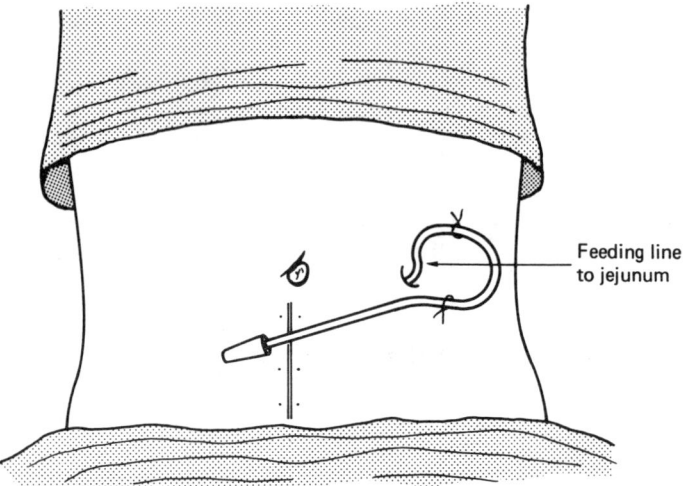

Figure 5.3 Feeding enterostomy after gastric surgery. It is possible to place a feeding tube in the stomach by percutaneous puncture.

Thus it is wise to keep prepared solutions in the refrigerator and to use them in 500 ml batches.

Feeds may be given by simple gravity infusion or by an enteral feeding pump. Pumps are useful because they save nursing time and, with a suitable halter to carry the apparatus, it is easier to mobilize the patient.

Complications of tube feeding

Nausea, abdominal distension and diarrhoea are the most common side-effects of enteral tube feeding. These symptoms can usually be reduced by controlling and reducing the flow of feed into the intestine. Troublesome diarrhoea is usually related to the previous use of broad-spectrum antibiotics or to small intestinal pathology. It is important to exclude drug-induced enteritis (especially pseudo-membranous colitis). Occasionally it may be necessary to give a small dose of codeine phosphate (30–60 mg t.d.s.) or of Imodium (up to 4 mg t.d.s.) for a few days.

Regurgitation and aspiration are potentially more serious side-effects. They occur particularly in patients with cerebral damage, in

Nutritional Support

those who have suffered severe trauma (e.g. road traffic accidents), in postoperative patients and in those with free gastro-oesophageal reflux, especially when this is associated with gastric atony. In such patients a Ryle's a tube should be used in the short term followed by direct feeding into the small intestine if the problem persists.

Metabolic complications of enteral nutrition are largely related to the underlying pathological disorder. Hyperglycaemia, electrolyte disturbances and abnormalities in the concentration of circulating hepatic enzymes are common. The infusion of 2000 kcal (8.4 MJ) a day may be excessive in some patients and this may contribute to impaired glucose tolerance and the tendency to fatty infiltration of the liver. None of these abnormalities appear to carry significant long-term sequelae so when discovered they should be managed at the time in their own right. Hypophosphataemia is an important complication which may occur as a result of the increased need for phosphorus in the patient metabolizing large quantities of carbohydrate (especially after a period of semistarvation) (see Table 3.10).

Laboratory monitoring

Patients' progress should be monitored carefully (Table 5.7). Daily weighing is a helpful indication of fluid retention (or losses) and over a period will give an indication of body mass. Urine should be tested daily for the presence or absence of glucose and a 24 h collection taken when there is doubt about nitrogen balance.

In the early phase of enteral feeding it is helpful to have a full blood count and measurement of circulating electrolytes, calcium, phosphate and magnesium twice a week. Liver function tests and circulating proteins should be estimated weekly. Anthropometric indices (measured monthly) are helpful in following the progress of some patients (arm muscle circumference, skin fold thickness and grip strength) (Table 5.8).

If the patient is receiving adequate quantities of minerals and vitamins (including folic acid) then routine measurements of iron, zinc, folic acid, ascorbic acid and vitamin B12 are unnecessary.

TOTAL PARENTERAL NUTRITION (TPN)

TPN is necessary when the patient requires nutritional support and the gastrointestinal tract is unavailable. The decision to use TPN should not be undertaken lightly. It is an expensive form of treatment (£50–

Table 5.7 Monitoring nutritional progress

Baseline
    Body weight (Ideal weight: usual weight)
    Anthropometric indices
    Full blood count
    Blood urea, creatinine, Na, K, (Cl), HCO_3
    Ca, Mg, P, alkaline phosphatase
    Iron TIBC, (Ferritin), Folate, B12
    Proteins
    Glucose, cholesterol, triglycerides
    Liver enzymes
Tests during period of stabilisation
    Daily
        Body weight
        Fluid intake/output. If electrolyte status uncertain test urine for Na, K
        Urine for sugar (or blood glucose)
        Electrolytes
Tests during prolonged care in hospital
    Daily
        Body weight
        Fluid intake/output
    Twice a week
        Urea and electrolytes
        Urine for sugar (or blood glucose)
    Once a week
        Full blood count
        Ca, Mg, phosphate
        Proteins
    Once a month
        Full baseline
Additional tests for those requiring long-term TPN
    Tests of vitamin and trace element status

100/day) and without meticulous care it may be hazardous. The indications for TPN are often not absolute. If there is doubt, a trial of enteral feeding may be helpful; if intravenous nutritional support is needed for only a few days then feeding via a peripheral vein is usually satisfactory.

At the other end of the scale long-term TPN (home parenteral nutrition) may have to be considered for the patient with intestinal failure. Such patients are best managed by a Specialist Regional Unit. At present in the UK no more than 1–2 per million population are maintained at home by total parenteral nutrition.

Table 5.8 *Anthropometry in monitoring the nutritional progress of a patient on long-term artificial enteral feeding*

Case: Mr A.B. 60 years old. Post intestinal resection—previously intensive care. Marked weight loss and weakness. Ideal weight 80 kg.

	Assessment	Follow-up (enteral tube feeding)	
	2/2/1988	6/3/1988	5/4/1988
Weight	62 kg	66 kg	68 kg
Skinfold			
Triceps	14 mm	16 mm	14 mm
Biceps	8 mm	8 mm	8.5 mm
Upper arm			
Circumference	29 cm	30 cm	30 cm
Muscle area	49 cm	50 cm	53 cm
Grip strength (mean 3 readings)	9.7 kg	15.7 kg	21.7 kg

Note: the grip strength in males (aged 20–65) ranges from 30–60 kg and in females (aged 20–65) from 20–40 kg. In this patient the expected grip strength in health was 50–55 kg.

Assessing requirements of the patient requiring TPN

The absolute requirements for intravenous nutrition include:

1. Fuels of respiration (principally carbohydrate and fat) for the production of energy-rich phosphate bonds (required for external work and for maintaining cellular integrity).
2. Amino acids for protein synthesis.
3. Salt and water to preserve intra- and extracellular hydration.
4. Essential fatty acids, cofactors, minerals and trace elements for cell structure and function.

For healthy subjects these requirements are reasonably well-defined (Table 5.9) but there are several imponderables. For example, there are few hard data regarding the correct amounts of trace elements and vitamins. This may be of little importance in short-term feeding but may be of considerable significance for the occasional patient requiring maintenance TPN for months.

TPN by-passes two important controls – the intestinal mucosa and

Table 5.9 Guide to baseline nutritional requirements for an adult requiring artificial nutrition

Nitrogen	8–12 g
Energy	1200–2000 kcals (5.0–8.4 MJ)
Electrolytes	
Sodium	70–150 mmol
Potassium	50–100 mmol
Chloride	70–220 mmol
Calcium	5–15 mmol
Magnesium	5–20 mmol
Phosphate	20–60 mmol (very variable)
Trace elements	
Iron	50 µmol
Zinc	100 µmol
(plus traces of chromium, copper, manganese, molybdenum, selenium, vanadium, iodide and fluoride)	
Vitamins	
B group in milligram quantities	
Thiamin 1.5, Riboflavin 2.5, Pyridoxine 2.5, Nicotinamide 15, Pantothenic acid 15, Biotin 0.5)	
B12	3 µg
Folic acid	0.5 mg
Ascorbic acid	20–50 mg
Retinol	1000 IU
Calciferol	5–15 µg
Tocopherol	5–15 µg

the liver. The metabolic effects of feeding nutrients directly into the systemic circulation are not fully understood as illustrated by a consideration of the divalent cations. Body iron status is normally controlled by absorptive mechanisms. Infusing large quantities of iron readily causes iron overload. Body calcium, magnesium and zinc are less tightly controlled by intestinal function but TPN may affect metabolic pathways. As a result hypercalciuria, hypercalcaemia and an unusual form of metabolic bone disease may occur in immobilized patients who require long-standing TPN. Again maintaining optimal concentrations of circulating magnesium and zinc is not always easy and during the early phase of refeeding hypophosphataemia may be a problem.

Thus special care must be exercised with patients who have metabolic disorders or who are unstable with respect to fluid and electro-

Nutritional Support

lytes. For the patient with excessive fluid losses it is usually easier to maintain the correct balance by infusing water and electrolytes through a peripheral line (in addition to the central-line feeding) rather than repeatedly to modify the TPN formula.

In practice, it is a useful clinical exercise to try to estimate the patient's needs on the basis of his present condition and his perceived metabolic requirements (Fig. 5.4). Nevertheless for most patients it is possible to use a standard regimen (Table 5.10). Patients rarely need TPN for more than a month, during which time the main aim is to keep the body functioning as well as possible.

MEETING REQUIREMENTS BY THE INTRAVENOUS ROUTE

The requirements of TPN may be met by using any one of a number of commercial preparations. Most large hospitals have developed standard protocols following discussions between interested clinicians and the hospital pharmacist. The underlying principles are as follows.

Sources of energy

Cellular energy is derived principally from glucose, fatty acids and some amino acids (via two carbon fragments and the tricarboxylic acid cycle).

Carbohydrates

Glucose is the carbohydrate of choice. It is cheap and readily assimilated, blood levels are easily monitored and when necessary are easily controlled by the judicious use of insulin. Fructose, sorbitol and xylitol offer no metabolic advantages and are prone to cause lactic acidosis, hyperuricaemia and hepatic dysfunction.

The glycolytic pathway provides a rate of oxidation of approximately 5 mg glucose/kg body weight/min, or approximately 1750 kcal (7.3 MJ)/day for a 70 kg man. Although it is possible to cover energy requirements using glucose alone there are disadvantages. Glucose at a high concentration is irritant to veins and if the rate of oxidation is exceeded the patient may develop hyperosmolar cellular dehydration.

Estimation of Energy and

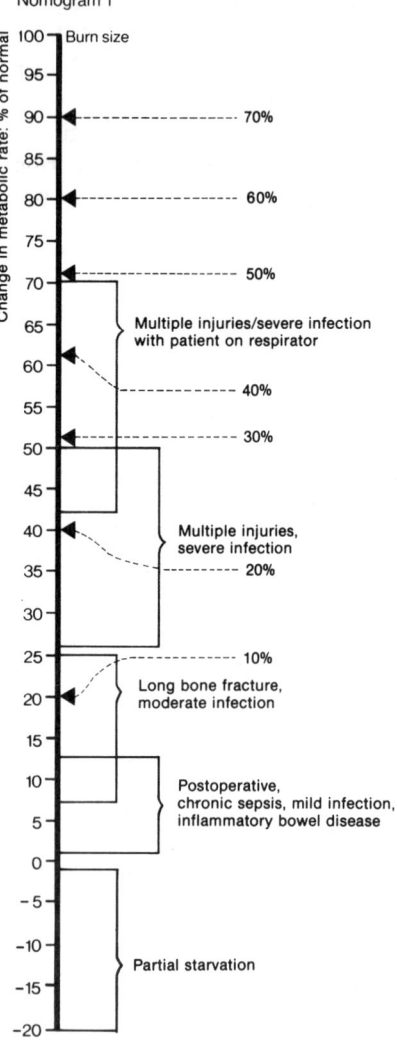

Nomogram 1

Weight		Basal Metabolic Rate (MR)	
kg	(lb)	kcal/day	(MJ/day)
30	(66)	850	(3.5)
35	(77)	950	(3.9)
40	(88)	1050	(4.3)
45	(99)	1150	(4.7)
50	(110)	1200	(5.1)
55	(121)	1300	(5.5)
60	(132)	1400	(5.8)
65	(143)	1450	(6.2)
70	(154)	1550	(6.5)
75	(165)	1650	(6.9)
80	(176)	1700	(7.2)
85	(187)	1800	(7.5)
90	(198)	1850	(7.8)
95	(209)	1950	(8.1)
100	(220)	2000	(8.4)
105	(231)	2100	(8.8)
110	(242)	2150	(9.1)

1. *Determine basal M.R.* for a normal person of that weight.

2. *Determine Energy Requirements*
   a) *Adjust* basal MR for stress (Nomogram 1)
   b) *Adjust* MR (stress) for 24 hour energy expenditure
   +20% 'Immobile'
   +30% Bed bound but mobile
   +40% Mobile in ward
   c) *Add* up to 1000 kcal/day extra if increase in energy stores is required. *Reduce* energy intake if loss of excess fat is required.

Nutritional Support

Nitrogen Requirements

Nomogram 2

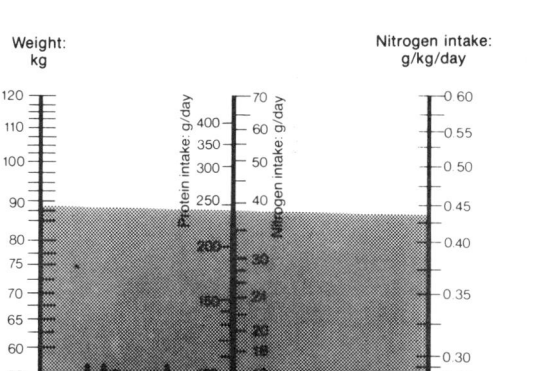

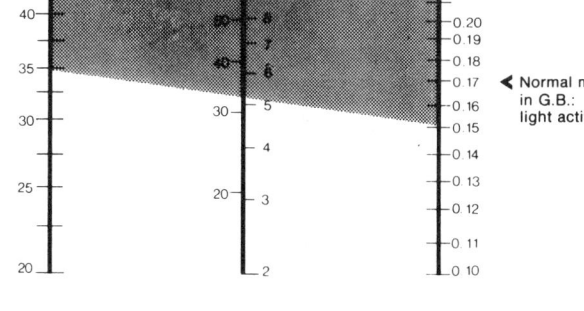

Figure 5.4 Table and nomogram for estimating energy and nitrogen requirements. (Reproduced by kind permission of Dr M. Elia, Dunn Nutrition Unit, Addenbrooke's Hospital, Cambridge and Travenol Limited.)

Table 5.10 Standard regimens for total parenteral nutrition

With all these regimens the bag is made up to contain 2 l of fluid in which there is 12.8 g nitrogen as amino acids, 90 mmol sodium, 110 mmol chloride, 7.5 mmol calcium, 7.5 mmol magnesium, 80 mmol potassium, 30 mmol phosphate and either 200 or 300 g of glucose.
In addition 500 ml of 5% or 10% lipid emulsion are provided.

	Standard		Standard low carbohydrate		High energy		Low energy	
	kcal	MJ	kcal	MJ	kcal	MJ	kcal	MJ
Total	2010	8.4	2060	8.6	2460	11.0	1610	6.7
CHO	1200	5.0	800	3.4	1200	5.0	800	3.4
Fat	550	2.3	1000	4.2	1000	4.2	550	2.3
CHO : FAT	2.2:1		0.73:1		1.1:1		1.4:1	
Cal : N(g)	157		169		200		126	

Additives (given alternate days—avoids interaction between trace elements and vitamins)

Vitamins		Trace elements	
A	10000 IU	Chromium	0.4 μmol
B		Copper	32 μmol
Thiamin	40 mg	Iron	40 μmol
Riboflavin	6.3 mg	Manganese	17 μmol
Pyridoxine	12.4 mg	Zinc	100 μmol
Niacin	100 mg		
Pantothenate	25 mg	Fluoride	120 μmol
Folic acid	15 mg	Iodide	2.4 μmol
C			
Ascorbate	500 mg		

Monthly injections
Vitamin B12 100 μg, Vitamin K 10 mg
(Vitamin D if no sunlight)

(From: Allwood M. C., McHutchinson D., Elia M. (1984). *A Guide to the Operation of a TPN Service.* Travend Laboratories, Egham, Surrey.)

Lipids

Long-chain triglycerides provide the alternative source of energy. Glycerol is converted to glucose to enter the glycolytic pathway and free fatty acids may be oxidized after crossing mitochondrial membranes. Alternatively, the fatty acids may be converted to ketone bodies which in turn can be used as a fuel for respiration.

In addition to providing calories, intravenous lipid preparations

Nutritional Support

contain essential fatty acids (linoleic, linolenic and arachidonic acids) which are needed for the synthesis of cell membranes. Lipid preparations are non-irritant and provide a high energy yield in a small volume with little disturbance of plasma osmolality. They are, however, expensive and hyperlipidaemia may occur in patients with impaired clearance mechanisms. Alternative fuels of lipid origin include medium-chain triglycerides, short-chain fatty acids and glycerol acetoacetate. These do not seem to offer any significant advantage.

Choice of fuel

A mixture of carbohydrate:fat (approximately 50:50) provides the most effective nitrogen-sparing regimen under most circumstances. There are data to suggest that the infusion of glucose alone is more effective in hypermetabolic patients but the picture in this respect is not completely clear. In practice, in most patients it is usual to give carbohydrate as the main source of energy because lipid is so expensive. A complete bottle of 10% lipid emulsion (Intralipid, Kabivitrum) gives 550 kcals (2.3 MJ) and 20% lipid emulsion 1000 kcals (4.2 MJ). It is reasonable to choose to give either no lipid or whole bottles of either 10% or 20% emulsion. The balance of calories is then made up with glucose (see Table 5.10). If it is decided to maintain the patient solely on glucose and amino acids then the body's requirements for essential fatty acids may be met by infusing the equivalent of 1 l of 20% lipid emulsion once a week.

Nitrogen

Amino acid requirements are less clearly defined than the number of calories. After major trauma and in severe illnesses some wasting of body protein is inevitable. The optimum amount of nitrogen to limit the negative nitrogen balance is difficult to estimate. The excretion of nitrogen in the urine is a good marker of body losses (see Chapter 3, p. 54) but this nitrogen is a combination of catabolized tissue protein and deaminated infused amino acids. Augmenting the infusion of amino acids may do no more than increase the excretion of nitrogen in the urine.

All solutions contain adequate amounts of the known essential amino acids. In malnourished subjects and those under stress, transamination may be relatively inefficient rendering non-essential amino acids semi-essential. Branched chain amino acids (valine leucine isoleucine) may have a specific effect on protein synthesis and under some circumstances appear to be as effective as a full mixture in reversing the negative nitrogen balance of surgical trauma.

The optimal amount and most appropriate mix of amino acids remains unresolved. Amino acids are metabolized by:

1. Incorporation into protein (either with or without transamination).
2. Deamination with conversion of ammonia to urea and of the carbon chain to glucose or keto acids.

Deamination is wasteful. Energy is better provided as carbohydrate or lipid both of which have a protein sparing effect. An active adult normally takes between 180 and 240 kcal (750 kJ and 1000 kJ)/g dietary nitrogen. For a patient in hospital the ratio should be lower because of the reduction in physical activity and the increased nitrogen needs to offset catabolic losses. Arbitrarily a ratio of 120–180 kcal/g nitrogen is usually accepted.

In practice it is sufficient to calculate approximate needs for nutrients (see Fig. 5.4) and then to provide an appropriate solution which in most cases can be taken from one of the standard regimens (see Table 5.10). Nitrogen, 12–13 g/day, will cover the amino acid requirements of most adults who are not seriously hypercatabolic. Thus in most cases it is necessary only to consider the most appropriate calorie intake and the tolerance to carbohydrate. Severely hypercatabolic patients may require additional nitrogen. The metabolic status of such patients should be carefully monitored.

Water and electrolytes

For most adult patients 2–3 l of fluid/day is appropriate. This should contain adequate sodium (60–100 mmol), potassium (60–90 mmol), calcium (5–15 mmol), magnesium (5–15 mmol), zinc (50 μmol), ferric iron 50–100 (μmol) and other trace elements; together with chloride (100–200 mmol), phosphate (20–80 mmol) and traces of iodide and fluoride. If there are constant additional losses (e.g. from a T-tube in the common bile duct) it may be possible to cover requirements by increasing the amount of electrolytes infused (Table 5.11) in unstable situations, however, it is better to rely on a separate peripheral infusion

Nutritional Support

Table 5.11 *Electrolyte losses in secretions*

Secretions	Electrolyte concentrations (mmol/l)			
	Na	K	Cl	HCO_3
Gastric	60	10	90	–
Pancreatic	140	5	75	90
Biliary	140	5	100	35
Small intestinal	100	15	100	25
Diarrhoea	60	30	45	45
Faeces	25	55	12	25

for close control of fluid and electrolyte status. In all cases this needs to be carefully monitored on a daily basis until the patient's requirements are clearly established. With prolonged TPN the possibility of trace element deficiency should be considered every 3 or 4 months. Departments of clinical biochemistry may have to enlist the aid of regional or supraregional services to provide adequate monitoring of trace element status.

Vitamins

The body has poor reserves of water-soluble vitamins (except vitamin B12) and thus these must be provided two or three times a week. There are good stores of fat-soluble vitamins (A, D, E) but vitamin K deficiency may occur as a result of reduced production by colonic bacteria (effect of antibiotics) and malabsorption. The requirements for vitamin D are best met by sunlight on the skin. This can be difficult to arrange and during long-term TPN it may be necessary to give vitamin D parenterally.

DELIVERY SYSTEMS

Nutrients are best delivered from a system which requires to be changed no more than once a day. The pharmacist prepares the day's solution by adding appropriate solutions to a 3-litre bag using a scrupulous aseptic technique. Many centres mix all nutrients together. Others prefer to infuse the lipid solution separately over the first 8 h. This allows nursing staff to check the clarity of the electrolyte –

carbohydrate solution and clinicians to ensure that the infused lipid is adequately cleared from the circulation.

If the pharmacy is unable to provide a service for the filling of 3-litre bags then solutions may be bought from a commercial compounding unit or given via a three container system which allows nitrogen and energy to be given simultaneously and electrolytes to be infused according to requirements (see Table 5.9).

Method of infusion

TPN is best delivered to the superior vena cava via a silastic catheter inserted by the intraclavicular approach into the subclavian vein tunnelled on the anterior chest wall (Fig. 5.5) where the skin surface is flat and relatively immobile. The catheterization should be performed by an experienced operator under aseptic conditions preferably in an operating theatre. After insertion of the catheter the skin site should be sprayed with a protective film, and covered with a semi-permeable adhesive dressing. A nurse experienced in the care of central lines should take responsibility for changing infusions and for dressing the catheter entry site (Table 5.12).

Before commencing TPN the line must be carefully checked for position (by chest x-ray) and patency (by lowering the infusion bottle to allow backflow). The described complications of catheter insertion are considerable and some are life-threatening. Most are completely avoidable (Table 5.13). TPN may be delivered by volumetric pump or allowed to flow in by gravity. Volumetric pumps work well but are expensive. Gravity feeding with a drip controller (e.g. IMED) provides almost as good a system, and slowing of the drip rate may give an early warning that the end of the line is becoming 'sticky'.

COMPLICATIONS OF TPN

Mechanical problems

The day-to-day care of a well-established TPN feeding line is usually remarkably trouble-free but the clinician must remain alert for possible complications (Table 5.14). Mechanical problems occur from time to time and when solving these care must be taken not to contaminate the line nor to allow air into the system. The patient's weight, urine output, circulating urea and electrolytes, urine and blood sugar should be

Nutritional Support

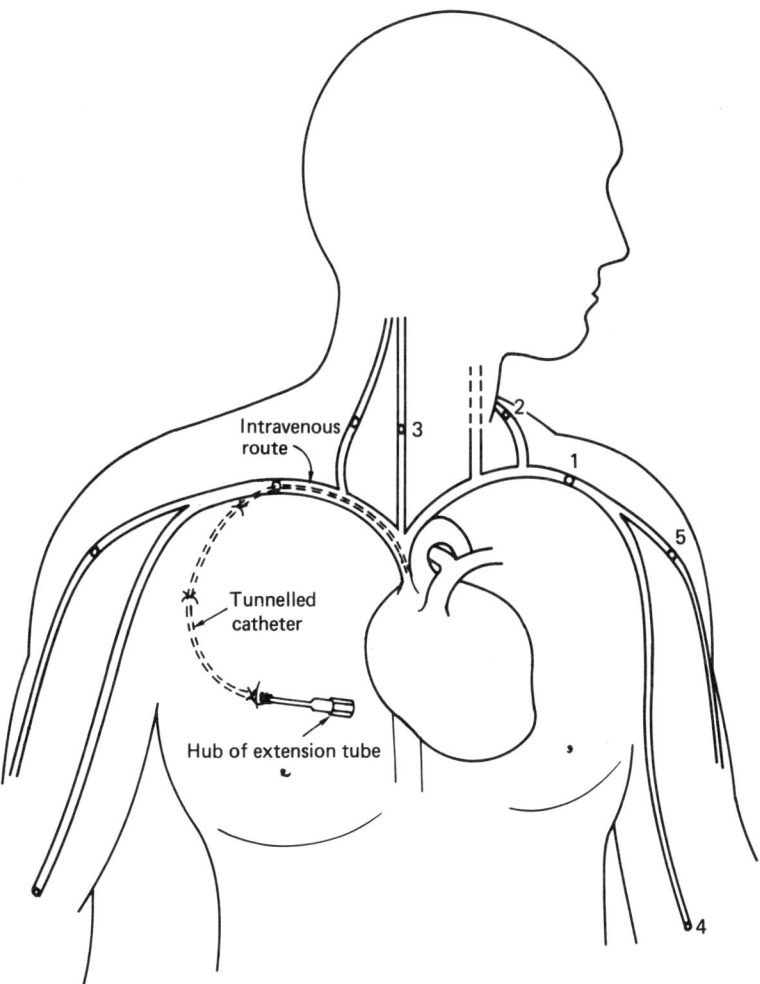

Figure 5.5 Points for insertion of a central venous catheter.
1 = Subclavian vein
2 = External jugular vein
3 = Internal jugular vein
4 = Basilic vein
5 = Cephalic vein

Table 5.12 *Care of central venous line for TPN*

Responsibility of trained nurse
   Dress catheter site (as indicated)
   Change infusion line under aseptic conditions
   Check and adjust flow rate
Responsibility of ward staff
   Monitor progress
   Protect line (never to be used for other purposes)
   Contact nutrition team if problems

Table 5.13 *Complications of catheter insertion*

Insertion trauma
  Arterial puncture (haematoma)
  Pneumothorax
  Haemothorax
  Nerve injury
Misplaced line
  Jugular vein—Thrombosis
  Right heart—Dysrhythmia, valve vegetation, perforation —tamponade
  Pleural cavity—Intrapleural infusion
Broken line
  Migration to right heart or pulmonary artery
Line dysfunction
  Air embolism
  Central venous thrombosis (tip incorrectly placed, poor flow with deposit of fibrin)

checked daily until the patient's condition is stable. Special care must be taken with patients who have renal, hepatic or cardiac failure, and usually the detailed management of such patients will be undertaken by an experienced member of staff.

Pyrexia is the main source of worry. In practice, during the first 2 weeks a carefully inserted and properly cared for feeding catheter is almost never the cause of focal infection. Immediately after surgery a low grade pyrexia is common and often can be ignored. At a later phase it is necessary to find the cause. An appropriate sequence of action might be as follows:

Table 5.14 *Mechanical problems with TPN lines*

Problem	Immediate action	Further action (Nutrition team)
Inconstant flow rate	Check mechanical system	Check catheter position Assess resistance to flow Clean catheter (urokinase)
Line leak	Check connection	Assess cause and change equipment (full sterile procedure)
Disconnection —air in line	Head-down tilt Clamp line	Check cause Clear line Reconnect
Bag empty	Maintain with slow infusion of saline	
Drip stops	Seek cause	Usually mechanical May need to clean catheter
Pyrexia	Seek cause Appropriate cultures Treat focal sepsis	Check line and skin tunnel Discuss need to remove line (Rarely urokinase and antibiotics via TPN line)

1. Examine the patient clinically (remember the possibility of deep vein thrombosis).
2. Look for signs of postoperative sepsis in a hidden site, e.g. subphrenic or pelvic abscess.
3. Culture appropriate specimens (e.g. sputum, urine, wound discharge).
4. Culture venous blood.
5. Arrange appropriate scans (especially chest x-ray).
6. Obtain total and differential white cell count.

If a specific cause for the pyrexia is not found most clinicians prefer to remove a 'probably infected' line and certainly this should be done if the skin tunnel becomes inflamed. Following the removal of an infected line the pyrexia usually settles promptly. Nevertheless tissue or metastatic infection may occur and the clinician must be prepared to treat systemically with antibiotics or antifungal agents.

In the occasional case with a particularly precious TPN line, it may be possible to clear the line of fibrin with urokinase and to eradicate low grade infection with an infusion of antibiotics. This decision should be made by an experienced clinician.

Metabolic problems

Side-effects from inappropriate infusions occur quite frequently (Table 5.15). Disorders of hydration are most common and are easily

Table 5.15 *Metabolic complications of TPN*

Metabolic disturbance	Precipitating factors
Extra-cellular fluid	
Overload	Cardiac, renal, hepatic failure
Hyperosmolar dehydration	Excess glucose, diabetes
Acid-base	
Hyperchloraemia	Rarely caused by TPN unless fructose or
Lactic acid	ethanol infused
Glucose	
Hyperglycaemia	Latent diabetes
Hypoglycaemia	Postinfusion high insulin
Lipid	
Hyperlipidaemia	Type IV diathesis
Fatty liver	Glucose in excess of needs
	Fat calories >CHO calories
EFA deficiency	Fat-free regimens for several weeks
Nitrogen	
Azotaemia	Renal insufficiency
Altered cerebration (headaches)	Too rapid infusion amino acids
Cholestatic hepatitis	Possibly amino acid induced
Minerals	
Hypokalaemia	During 'flow' phase of injury
Hypocalcaemia	Inadequate provision (check vitamin D and magnesium)
Hypomagnesaemia	Inadequate provision (usually in face of excess losses)
Hypophosphataemia	Carbohydrate infusions with insufficient phosphate
Metabolic bone disease	Cause uncertain

recognized if the patient is weighed daily. Overfeeding sick patients is also a common error. Obsessional concern with increasing or at least maintaining body weight may cause hyperglycaemia, hyperlipidaemia, hepatic congestion (with glycogen and water) and a high respiratory quotient with the conversion of glucose to fat. Excess nitrogen may

Nutritional Support

exacerbate renal failure and disturb cerebral function (headache is a not uncommon symptom with over-rapid infusion of amino acids).

Deficiency syndromes occasionally occur in patients undergoing prolonged intravenous feeding (Table 5.16). These are difficult to

Table 5.16 *Total parenteral nutrition—vitamin and trace element deficiencies*

Trace element	Effects of deficiency
Biotin	Hair loss, eczematous dermatitis, depression
Chromium	Glucose intolerance, neuropathy
Copper	Anaemia, neutropaenia
Folate	Pancytopaenia
Selenium	Myalgia, cardiomyopathy
Zinc	Peristomal and acral dermatitis

guard against because there is no simple way of assessing nutritional status with respect to vitamins, minerals and trace elements.

Monitoring progress

The mode of monitoring the progress of patients on TPN is similar to that for enteral feeding (see Table 5.7). It is important, however, to remember that progress is usually much more turbulent. Firstly the patients are often sick and may require the sort of attention provided in an intensive care unit. Secondly, with TPN, the intestine and liver can no longer provide 'first pass' control. The opportunity for doing harm is considerable and patients are often consciously or subconsciously aware that their body has lost an important physiological control. They should be given the chance to voice their fears and offered as much psychological support as can be given.

The changeover to enteral feeding should take place over 3 or 4 days giving the body as a whole, and the gut in particular, time to adjust. Usually there is little difficulty.

HOME PARENTERAL NUTRITION

Long-term TPN is technically feasible. At present about 50 patients in the UK are being maintained by this form of treatment. The indications and management of home TPN are outside the scope of this book. Nevertheless in most cases patients and their relatives cope extremely well given the support of a specialized team. Catheter-related sepsis is not common and well-selected patients lead a full and active life (one woman in the North of England has had two children during her life on TPN).

THE NUTRITION TEAM

Several large hospitals have demonstrated the value of having a nutrition team to advise and coordinate the management of patients requiring nutritional support. The team should be able to standardize regimens, to rationalize the use of equipment and to teach ward staff. Usually a specialist nurse is the key member. She is responsible for ensuring standards of care for patients on TPN, organizing seminars for nursing staff and maintaining the records of the nutrition team. The team itself may include:

A consultant clinician with an interest in clinical nutrition.
A clinical registrar/senior registrar to cope with day-to-day problems.
A senior pharmacist to decide how best to meet nutritional requirements in patients requiring TPN and to advise on the addition of drugs to TPN solutions if this makes for easier management.
A senior dietitian to advise on enteral nutrition and diets for the severely malnourished.
A clinical biochemist to assist with monitoring the progress of patients.
A specialist nurse to provide the organization that ensures the highest standards of care.

The actual structure and function of the team will vary from hospital to hospital. It may be appropriate to include an intensive therapy unit specialist, an anaesthetist (skilled in the insertion of central venous catheters), a ward sister (who may provide a base for the team), a physiotherapist (with a special interest in mobilizing the patient on TPN) and a social worker (if the unit has a heavy commitment to patients receiving TPN at home).

The management of nutritional support for the acutely sick is a challenge to ward clinicians. The meeting of this challenge should lead to a situation in which patients with treatable chronic disorders are not allowed to become malnourished.

FURTHER READING

Diets

Russell R., ed. (1983). *Elemental Diets*. London: Academic Press.

Nutritional support

Silk D. B. A. (1983). *Nutritional Support in Clinical Practice*. Oxford: Blackwell Scientific Publications.
Wilmore D. W. (1977). *Metabolic Management of the Critically Ill*. New York: Plenum Press.

Enteral and parenteral nutrition

Jeejeebhoy K. N. (1983). *Total Parenteral Nutrition in the Hospital and at Home*. Boca Raton, Florida: CRC Press Inc.
Rombeau J. L., Caldwell M. D., eds. (1984). *Enteral and Tube Feeding*. Philadelphia: W. B. Saunders Co.
Rombeau J. L., Caldwell M. D., eds. (1986). *Parenteral Nutrition*. Philadelphia: W. B. Saunders Co.

Chapter

6

Diet and the Epidemiology of Disease

GENERAL PRINCIPLES • CHOLESTEROL AND FAT • SALT • FIBRE AND REFINED CARBOHYDRATE • REFINED SUGAR • ALCOHOL • FURTHER READING

GENERAL PRINCIPLES

The effect of diet on the health of populations excites enormous interest and controversy. Thus observations based on the extraordinary variations in the geographical distribution of cancer has led to a detailed examination of possible associations with diet (Table 6.1). Many disorders, common in affluent societies, appear not to afflict the ordinary people of the developing world. Again diet may be an important determining factor (Table 6.2). Clinicians must be sensibly aware of the possibilities of disease caused by diet and be able to advise their patients. There is no doubt that the opinions of the medical profession influence public attitudes and behaviour. For example, although difficult to quantitate, the medical profession has played a major part in reducing the prevalence of smoking in the UK. With diet, however, doctors should be cautious in making pronouncements. It is difficult to demonstrate conclusively that ordinary diets cause disease. Much of the evidence is epidemiological. The aetiology of most common conditions is multifactorial with many interacting variables including genetic inheritance, social background, living conditions, personality, stress, exercise, and personal habits, such as smoking and the drinking of alcohol. It is difficult to control the many independent variables and thus it is easy to contest the epidemiological data. Furthermore, intervention studies are difficult to design and carry out

Table 6.1 Associations of diet with cancer

Site of cancer	Geography	Dietary association
Buccal mucosa	South-east Asia South-east Africa Puerto Rico	Chewing plants (e.g. betal nut, tobacco)
Oesophagus	Southern and eastern Africa Caspian Sea area	Maize beer Poor diet—low in fruit/vegetables
Stomach	Japan Chile/Colombia	Salty/pickled foods (negative association with vitamin C content)
Colon	Europe North America	Affluent diets with a high content of meat and fat and low content of fibre
Liver	Africa South-east Asia	Mainly hepatitis B Aflatoxin contaminated food
Breast	Europe North America	High fat intake correlates best
Lung	USA Japan Norway (Interestingly negative in the UK)	Low vitamin A (doubtful)

effectively, especially when there is a long latent period between putative cause and measurable effect.

For example, in the Multiple Risk Factor Intervention Trial for ischaemic heart disease (MRFIT study), 12 866 high risk men aged 35–57 years were randomly allocated either to a special intervention (SI) programme or to 'usual care' (UC). The intervention included treatment for hypertension, counselling for smoking and dietary advice aimed at lowering blood cholesterol. The subjects were observed for a mean of 7 years (not less than 6 years). The basic observations are shown in Table 6.3. Both groups had a considerably lower mortality than expected. This reduced the statistical power of the comparison. Moreover the investigators underestimated the effect of identifying patients at high risk and informing both them and their medical advisers of this risk. Thus UC had a greater effect on risk factors than

Table 6.2 *Disorders which may be, in part, determined by nutritional factors*

Disorder	Nutrient
Ischaemic heart disease	Fat
Colonic disorders	
Constipation	Fibre
Polyps and cancer	Fat/protein/fibre
Diverticular disease	Fibre
(Irritable bowel)	?Fibre
Metabolic diseases	
Obesity	Excess calories from refined food
Diabetes mellitus	
Vascular disease	
Hypertension	Salt
Varicose veins	
Deep venous thrombosis	?Fibre
Haemorrhoids	
Stone disease	
Gallstones	
Renal stones	?Affluent diet
Tooth decay	
Dental caries	Sticky foods (refined sugar)
Inflammatory disorders	
Appendicitis	?Fibre
Inflammatory bowel disease	No clear evidence
Allergic disorders	Some foods implicated, e.g. dairy produce, wheat, shellfish

expected. The mortality from ischaemic heart disease was only 7% higher than in the SI group. This difference was not significant.

Thus it seems that short-term studies are unlikely to answer the questions raised by epidemiological observations. Nevertheless the clinician cannot ignore matters which are of such great public concern. Unfortunately, but perhaps not surprisingly, advice on diet offered by the medical profession to the public and to governments has had a chequered history. In the 1930s, with sub-optimal nutrition prevalent in the poorer segments of the population, (as shown in the heights and weights of school children), the emphasis was on the provision of first class protein. Meat, milk, eggs and cheese were regarded as essential for optimal growth and development. The more the better. With an ample

Diet and the Epidemiology of Disease

Table 6.3 Data from the National Institutes of Health Multiple Risk Factor Intervention Trial for prevention of coronary heart disease*

Men aged 35–57 years free from clinical evidence of coronary heart disease (CHD), but with risk scores in the upper 10% (as defined by Framingham data) were recruited and followed for a mean of 7 years (minimum 6 years). Risk factors
  Serum cholesterol 250 mg or more
  Smoking 30 cigarettes or more a day
  Diastolic blood pressure >90 mmHg
Random assignment to groups
  Special intervention (SI)
  Usual care (UC)

	Number studied		CHD deaths		Total deaths	
	SI	UC	SI	UC	SI	UC
Total	4602	4670	68	88	171	185
BP normal	1817	1862	24	30	71	63
BP raised	2785	2808	44	58	100	122
Cholesterol						
<250	2061	2095	34	37	85	89
>250	2541	2575	34	51	86	96
Non-smokers	1692	1730	16	26	38	49
Smokers	2910	2940	52	62	133	136

*MRFIT Group. (1982). Multiple risk factor intervention trial: Risk factor changes and mortality results. *JAMA*; **248**: 1465–77.

diet based on first class protein, other nutritional requirements should take care of themselves (except for ascorbic acid, the needs for which it was suggested could be met by green leaves and citrus fruits).

After the war these attitudes persisted in spite of the obviously beneficial effects of food rationing in Britain between 1939 and 1945. Indeed the wartime diet would have met most of the 1983 recommendations of the National Advisory Committee on Nutrition Education (see Table 1.8). Meat, eggs, fats, cheese, sugar and milk were strictly rationed. Bread was made from low extraction flour, potatoes and vegetables (often home grown) were freely available. The poor got reasonable food at a price they could afford and the food industry had little opportunity to produce more than the simplest processed foods. There was no outbreak of disease due to dietary deficiency although medical advisors to the DHSS were concerned about the provision of vitamin C and vitamin D for infants. Concentrated orange juice and cod liver oil were provided free. Even this limited supplement carried hidden dangers leading to a minor epidemic of hypercalcaemia due to hypervitaminosis D. But overall the British were healthier than they had ever been.

Nevertheless, the concept of an overwhelming need for first class protein persisted. Dairy products and fattened animals had their heyday. Bread and potatoes were regarded as stodgy foods, twin evils in the development of obesity. The food industry concentrated on the development of easily prepared, highly palatable, processed foods with a long shelf life.

The problem

Throughout this century the pattern of disease has changed dramatically. Infection is no longer the main cause of mortality in the young and middle-aged. By the late 1920s heart attacks (coronary thrombosis) had become sufficiently common to produce discussion in medical journals. A decade later disorders of the heart and cardiovascular system overtook infectious disease as the most common cause of death. Today myocardial infarction accounts for a half of all male deaths in middle age (i.e. in the 20 years before retirement at 65). In the UK the probable role of a high intake of animal fat in the aetiology of ischaemic heart disease has been accepted only slowly. In the USA, a whole generation has been exposed to the pressures of health experts stimulated by a succession of reports starting in 1959 with that of the American Heart Association: *Dietary fat and its relationship to heart attacks and strokes.* (see Council on Foods and Nutrition, 1959.) It is probable that a change in diet has played its part in the fall of the death rate from ischaemic heart disease in American males from over 800 to less than 600/100 000 population (1968–1978). Over the same period, figures for England and Wales have shown a slight increase and now exceed those for the USA (Fig. 6.1).

The cholesterol controversy has tended to overshadow other possible dietary factors in the genesis of cardiovascular disease of which the intake of salt is perhaps the most important. Indeed, in 1979 a group of experts for the American Society of Clinical Nutrition (Symposium, 1979) stated that the correlation between salt intake and hypertension provided the clearest link between diet and 'disease of affluence'.

The other major nutrition debate concerns the possible relationship between dietary fibre and colonic disorders (extended rather tenuously to include a number of other pathologies; see Table 6.4). Fibre intake

Diet and the Epidemiology of Disease

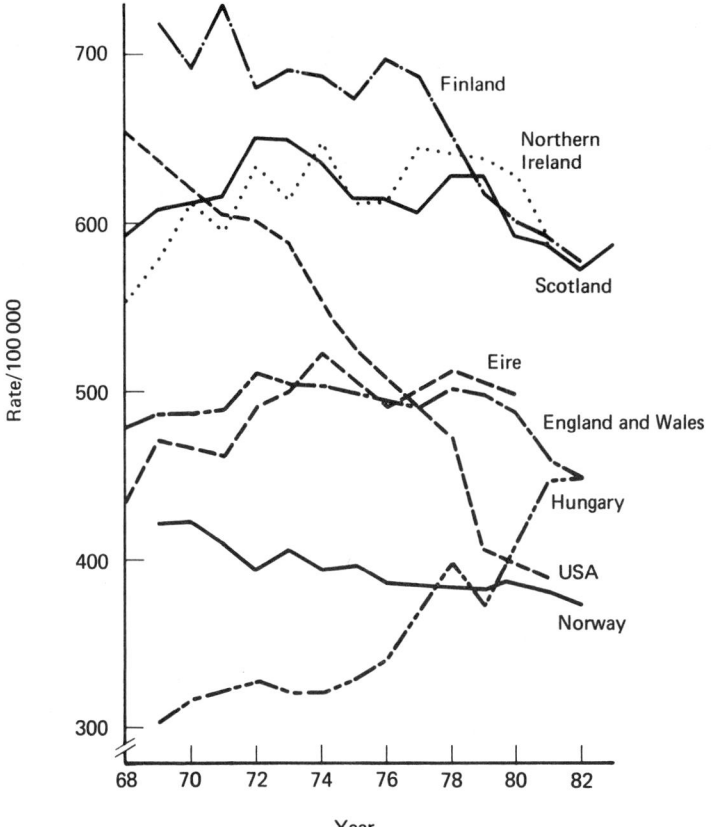

Figure 6.1 Trends in mortality rates in ischaemic heart disease in men aged 40–69. (Reproduced by kind permission of Professor H. Tunstall-Pedoe and the editor of the *Scottish Health Bulletin*.)

has been a central factor in this debate, although for cancer of colon the intake of animal fat and protein may be more important. If these associations between nutrition and both cardiovascular and gastro-intestinal disease are substantiated then the changes we see occurring in the national diet will accelerate (see Fig. 1.2). The nation will eat a diet containing less fat (especially less animal fat), more unrefined carbo-hydrate (with less refined sugar), less salt and less alcohol. The prudent

Table 6.4 Disorders which may be related to a low intake of dietary fibre

Colonic
  Appendicitis
  Irritable bowel
  Diverticulosis coli
  Colonic polyps
  Cancer of the colon
Metabolic
  Obesity
  Diabetes mellitus
  Gallstones
  Ischaemic arterial disease
Motility
  Constipation
  Hiatal hernia
  Piles
  Varicose veins

Possible effects of fibre on intestinal function
  Rate of transit
  Rate of uptake of nutrients (especially carbohydrates)
  Stool bulk
  Intestinal muscle activity
  Intestinal bacteriology
  Colonic absorption, especially soluble fatty acids, minerals and bile salts
  Absorption of intestinal toxins

diet will continue to contain 11% protein (a remarkably constant figure in affluent industrialized countries and one which has changed little this century), but it will be associated with less animal fat (i.e. skimmed rather than whole milk; cottage rather than hard cheese and lean rather than marbled meat). The clinician must be aware of the pressures mediating such important changes in the eating habits of the nation.

Thus the disorders of nutrient deficiency (excluding fibre) are no longer a general problem in Britain although certain groups remain at risk (e.g. vitamin deficiency in the elderly, rickets in the children of Asian immigrants). Overall the intake of food is probably excessive and the balance unsatisfactory. Finally the rising consumption of alcohol is a cause for concern.

Diet and the Epidemiology of Disease

Nutrient deficiency in Britain – community aspects

In the industrialized world few people suffer from the diseases of dietary deficiency. Some foods are fortified and in some cases this is undoubtedly beneficial. Iodide added to table salt prevents goitre and fluoridation of drinking water lessens the risk of dental caries. Vitamin D added to margarine and infant foods almost certainly reduces the incidence of rickets and osteomalacia (although this is now much less important as a result of the Clean Air Act and of the increased bodily exposure to sunlight). Nutrients are added to bread, cereals and cereal products including B group vitamins, calcium and iron. There is little evidence that these improve community health, although in the UK the fortification of flour with calcium undoubtedly provides an important dietary source of this mineral. In industrialized countries, iron deficiency is the only common nutritional deficiency but the availability of iron added to flour is low.

Fluoridation of water is the only nutritional additive which generates a public response. Control of the water supply is a responsibility of local government and despite repeated recommendations by the WHO, in many areas fluoridation is bitterly and successfully opposed for what appear to be emotional reasons. The addition of fluoride to toothpaste has to some extent circumvented opposition to mass 'medication' and may be the most important factor in decreasing the incidence of dental caries (see Fig. 6.2).

CHOLESTEROL AND FAT

Relationships with cardiovascular disease

Atheromatous disease is the most important health problem in Western society. The risk factors have been clearly identified (Table 6.5) but

Table 6.5 *Risk factors for ischaemic heart disease (IHD)*

Age	Obesity
Sex	Smoking
Genes	Lack of exercise
Stress	(Diet)
Hypercholesterolaemia	

their relative importance and inter-relationships are poorly understood. Until the pathogenesis of atheroma has been clearly established, doctors are unable to be dogmatic in giving dietary advice. Nevertheless the circumstantial evidence in favour of a significant role for circulating cholesterol is very considerable (see reports listed in Table 7.2). Unfortunately the subsidiary hypothesis that circulating cholesterol is a function of the intake of saturated fat and cholesterol is rather less secure, and much of the controversy about the role of diet turns on this debate (Table 6.6).50

Table 6.6 Role of dietary fat in ischaemic heart disease (IHD)

Histopathology	Content of atheromatous plaques Experimental studies in animals (but poor analogy with human disorder)
Genetic disease	Familial hypercholesterolaemia, ischaemic heart disease from childhood
Epidemiology	IHD correlates with circulating cholesterol between and within populations
Prospective studies	Many studies (>20) in affluent countries show hypercholesterolaemia, hypertension and smoking as major risk factors for IHD The Framingham Study (1980)* shows long incubation period
Retrospective studies	Changes in life style alter incidence of IHD (e.g. Japanese to USA)
Intervention studies	Decrease IHD but impossible to disentangle effects of reduced smoking, control of hypertension, increased exercise. Karelia (Finland), Mr Fit (USA)

*Dawber T. R. (1980). *The Framingham Study*: the epidemiology of atherosclerotic disease. (A Commonwealth Fund Book.) Cambridge, Massachusetts: Harvard University Press.

Certainly, intervention studies have shown that it is possible to reduce the incidence of ischaemic heart disease. So far, however, it has been impossible to prove that changes in diet are more important than the effect of other variables, such as increased exercise, reduced smoking, control of hypertension and improved care of diabetics. In the Framingham study the chances of a heart attack correlated significantly with the level of circulating cholesterol but not with diet. (Proponents of the dietary hypothesis suggest that the population

Diet and the Epidemiology of Disease 177

studied was taking too much animal fat to allow diet to be separated as an independent variable.) More worryingly, in adults it is difficult to reduce mean plasma cholesterol by more than 10% by dietary manipulation. The clinical benefit of treating an adult with a high cholesterol level is almost impossible to demonstrate. To date the benefits of lowering cholesterol levels have been proven only for men in the top 5% of the usual range and this has been achieved only by giving drugs in addition to modifying diet. Nevertheless, on the basis of epidemiological evidence the NIH Consensus Development Conference (1984) on cholesterol and heart disease concluded that diet should be modified to reduce blood cholesterol to 180 mg/dl (4.6 mmol/l) for adults under 30 and 200 mg/dl (5.1 mmol/l) for people over 30. It is believed that this may be achieved by a diet which maintains ideal body weight, with fat providing no more than 30% calories (saturated fat reduced to 10% calories) and containing less than 250–300 mg cholesterol. The sceptics raise doubts regarding the possible side-effects of applying dietary restriction universally – irrespective of age, sex or circulating cholesterol – and emphasize alternative means of lowering circulating cholesterol in those at risk (vegetarian diets, 'Mediterranean diets' high in monosaturated fats, 'Eskimo diets' containing fish oil). They also emphasize the need to understand the factors determining the low rates of coronary heart disease in developed countries like France and Japan.

At present the majority of cardiologists and scientists with an interest in atheroma favour a policy of national dietary intervention. The more cautious believe that scientists should do no more than provide scientifically sound conclusions and should state clearly the gaps in our knowledge. They would leave the policy-makers to come to their own conclusions. Inevitably these are biased by political, social and economic factors.

Over the last decade in the USA, Canada and Australia age-adjusted mortality from cardiovascular disease has fallen (see Fig. 6.1). This change has occurred against a background of a significant reduction in the prevalence of risk factors. The figures contrast quite strikingly with the lack of change or increase in death rates from heart attacks in developed countries where changes in human behaviour have been less marked (Germany, Denmark, Britain, eastern Europe). Nevertheless for better or worse a change in eating habits in the UK is already occurring particularly amongst the better educated, more affluent segments of the population. It will be interesting to watch mortality figures over the next decade or two, but important to recall that, in at least one intervention study, mortality from coronary heart disease has been associated with a reciprocal increase in deaths from other causes.

SALT

Relationships to hypertension

Salt as a factor in cardiovascular disease has received much less publicity than cholesterol and fat. Yet the importance of a high sodium intake in the genesis of hypertension has persuasive epidemiological backing. In Western society, where sodium intake is high, blood pressure rises more rapidly with age and hypertension is more common than in primitive societies which use little salt. The highest recorded incidence of hypertension is in northern Japan where individuals ingest more than 400 mmol sodium/day. In areas where the daily individual intake is less than 50 mmol/day hypertension is rarely found. The argument implicating salt is also supported to some extent by clinical observations. In hypertensive subjects the concentration of sodium in red cells is high and ionic transport across membranes is deranged. Reduction of body sodium lowers blood pressure more in subjects with hypertension than in those without. Conversely, an increase in dietary sodium is more likely to elevate the blood pressure of a hypertensive subject than in someone who is normotensive.

Further support comes from experimental studies. Hypertension can be produced in some laboratory animals by feeding them with sodium chloride. The tendency is genetically determined; some strains are salt-sensitive, others salt-resistant. Experimentally-induced hypertension does not produce atheroma *per se*, but it will accelerate the damage to arterial walls produced by atherogenic diets.

Despite these lines of evidence, the available data does not prove that salt intake is a prime determinant of hypertension. It is difficult to exclude the effects of other population variables. Genetic make-up, body weight, potassium intake, exercise and cultural habits may all be relevant to the development of hypertension. Scientists are uncertain whether or not dietary sodium controls the undoubted changes in sodium metabolism occurring in hypertensive subjects. A similar change may be found in their normotensive relatives or may appear as an epiphenomenon in patients with secondary hypertension (e.g. as a result of renal artery stenosis).

It has been suggested that up to 10% of human subjects may be genetically susceptible to essential hypertension and that a lifelong restriction of salt intake to less than 60 mmol/day could prevent the rise in blood pressure. Unfortunately, in established hypertension salt restriction causes only a modest and uneven fall in blood pressure. Nevertheless this change may be helpful in enhancing the effect of anti-hypertensive drugs. Loss of weight also leads to a fall in blood pressure and this change appears to operate independently of the effect of salt restriction.

Because of these reservations it is difficult to balance the likely benefits and disadvantages of a nationwide major reduction of salt intake. There are no extensive controlled trials of the long-term effects of a low salt diet. One may predict a low risk of adverse side-effects on the basis of the relatively recent introduction of added salt into human diets (a few thousand years at most) and the apparent absence of disorders due to sodium deficiency in tribes to whom salt is not readily available. Special care might have to be taken with pregnant women and the very few patients with salt-losing states, such as Addison's disease and salt-losing nephropathy.

It is difficult to know if the modest restriction of salt intake proposed by NACNE could be of benefit. Almost certainly it could not cause harm. If adopted widely it would give the food industry time to adapt to a demand for less salt in prepared foods. Food processing firms would have time to find other preservatives and to test these for hidden toxic effects which might be greater than those ascribed to sodium chloride.

Meanwhile there is a real need for a well-designed intervention trial. For example, it might be possible to test the effects of rigorous salt restriction on a large group of young people identified as carrying significant risk factors for essential hypertension (e.g. positive family history, high normal blood pressure in adolescence and a resting heart rate disproportionate to physical condition). Unfortunately, as with other dietary recommendations, the interested clinical scientist has to work firstly against a background of pronouncements by well-meaning but scientifically-naive publicists, and secondly in the face of active disinterest by central government and their advisers who find it difficult to ignore economic and political pressures.

FIBRE AND REFINED CARBOHYDRATE

Relationship with gastrointestinal pathology and related disorders

Gastrointestinal disease is common in industrialized countries. Since 1970 a low intake of fibre has been regarded as the main cause of colonic and related disorders. This idea was popularized primarily by Burkitt who added his observations on diseases in central Africa to those of Cleave (1969; 1974), Trowell (1981; 1985) and Walker (1971). They were impressed by the low incidence of appendicitis, diverticular disease, benign and malignant tumours of the colon and haemorrhoids in the developing countries; they thought that the different pattern of disease might be due to differences in diet, and in particular they drew attention to the much higher intake of fibre by people living in regions with a low incidence of colonic disease. Two aspects of diet have received special attention:

1. The amount of fibre in the diet.
2. The intake of refined carbohydrates (especially sucrose).

Cleave published his conclusions by emphasizing the role of excess refined sugar ('the saccharine disease'). Whereas Walker, Burkitt and Trowell concentrated on the lack of fibre.

The hypothesis was extended to cover disorders which may be related physically or biochemically to colonic function (see Table 6.4) and has become entwined with other possibly deleterious features of Western living, such as excess smoking, excess alcohol, insufficient exercise and an excess intake of animal fat and salt.

As with the merits of a diet high in first-class protein the medical profession has been far from consistent in its advice over fibre. Hippocrates recognized that unrefined cereals have a faecal bulking effect, and in the 19th century there were strong protagonists of their value in promoting health, especially Graham in the USA and Allinson in the UK. In fact, by expounding the virtues of wholemeal bread and criticizing contemporary medicines, Allinson infuriated the medical hierarchy so much that he was struck off the Medical Register. In the early 20th century, both in the UK (Arbuthnott Lane) and the USA (Alvarez), fermentation of colonic contents was believed to cause a variety of disorders by auto-intoxication. Alvarez was the leading gastroenterologist of the day and forcibly expressed the opinion that man as a carnivore should not eat extra roughage. Lane went further

Diet and the Epidemiology of Disease

and recommended colectomy for disorders as diverse as rheumatoid arthritis, diabetes mellitus and flat feet which he ascribed to autointoxication from chronic intestinal sepsis (see Lane, 1918). He had a large London practice and was the reputed model for Sir Cutler Walpole in Bernard Shaw's *Doctor's Dilemma*. Other authorities, including Kellogg (of cereal bran fame) and Hurst the (founder of British gastroenterology who wrote a treatise on the *Treatment of constipation and allied disorders*) expounded alternative views. They believed that mankind should have trouble-free bowel actions and that this could be best achieved by a high intake of wheat bran.

Constipation

There is no doubt that increasing the intake of fibre will increase faecal bulk and in most subjects lead to the more frequent passage of softer faeces. In hospital studies of elderly subjects, the provision of wholemeal bread and bran biscuits increased the frequency of bowel actions with few side-effects – just occasional flatulence or distension. Experimental data has shown that the action of an increased intake of fibre is most prominent in the least constipated and is more marked in men than in women. These features limit the use of fibre as a therapeutic agent. Nevertheless if the overall consumption of fibre were to increase it is reasonable to suppose that the national demand for aperients would decrease. The likely effect on the prevalence of bowel disorders other than constipation is much less certain.

Irritable bowel syndrome

Functional abdominal pain is very common in Western society. Mild attacks appear to affect most people from time-to-time, often against a background of intermittent constipation. Colonic spasm has been demonstrated both radiologically and by pressure studies. Spasm is believed not only to cause abdominal discomfort but also to lead to the development of colonic diverticula.

Increasing the amount of fibre in the diet accelerates slow transit and possibly slows rapid transit of material through the gut. Thus it is suggested that fibre acts as a regulator of intestinal motility. An increased intake of dietary fibre may help many patients with irritable bowel syndrome but in practice not all respond.

The interpretation of the effects of fibre on colonic function are confounded by observations on the Masai and on Eskimoes. These people eat diets containing virtually no fibre – in the one case meat and milk and in the other fish and sea mammals – yet pass small quantities of soft stool without difficulty.

The evidence that a high fibre diet will protect against other disorders listed in Table 6.4 (p. 174) is largely circumstantial. These conditions are seen rarely in developing countries and people migrating from low to high risk areas take on the disease patterns of their new environment. In industrialized countries, the average intake of dietary fibre of most people is less than a quarter of those eating African diets based on millet, rice and root vegetables. The hypothesis that constipation, irritable bowel, diverticular disease and haemorrhoids are closely related to the amount of fibre in the diet is largely dependent on these observations.

Diverticular disease

Colonic diverticulosis is found in 20% of British adults aged 50–60 years and in up to 40% of those aged 70–80 years. Diverticula probably do not cause symptoms without some complicating factor. Much so called diverticular disease is no more than an irritable bowel syndrome (spastic colon) in patients in whom the radiologist can demonstrate diverticula. Nevertheless diverticulitis, pericolonic inflammation and stricture formation are painful and distressing disorders best avoided. Diverticula are found less commonly in vegetarians (12%) than in control subjects (33%), an observation which offers support to the general theory. But in one study it was shown that vegetarians with diverticula in their colons eat rather less fibre than those without! It is now usual to ask patients with spasmodic abdominal pain and colonic diverticula to add bran to their diet. Early reports claimed very significant benefits for such patients and a fall in the rate of diverticular complications. Certainly patients with hard stools become less constipated and sometimes those with diarrhoea are also relieved of their symptoms. But residual abdominal discomfort is common and from recent studies it is clear that fibre is not a universal panacea for the ills of people with colonic diverticulosis. Indeed some subjects appear to be intolerant of wheat bran and their symptoms are exacerbated.

Diet and the Epidemiology of Disease

Cancer of the colon

Across the world the incidence of cancer of the colon varies 20-fold with high figures in the British Isles (especially Ireland and Scotland) and very low figures in the countries of central and east Africa. Japan is the only industrialized country with a relatively low incidence (approximately one-third of that of the USA and the UK) and Japanese moving to the West take on the pattern of pathology of the host country. The geographical variations and the study of special groups within countries (e.g. vegetarians) suggest that environment is an important factor in the development of large bowel cancer. Nevertheless epidemiological data linking large bowel cancer with diet are confusing. Overall there appear to be positive correlations with high intakes of meat, fat, sugar, eggs and total calories. Theories have been advanced to support links with high intakes of protein, fat and cholesterol and with a low intake of fibre. It is suggested that fibre acts by diluting carcinogens in stools through its bulking action and by increasing the rate of clearance of potentially harmful bacterial metabolites, such as the dehydroxylated bile acids.

In general there are some grounds to support the statement that in susceptible people a high fibre diet reduces the risk of large bowel cancer. If this diet is based on unprocessed foods with a high content of carbohydrate then it will also be low in fat, cholesterol and animal protein.

The average British diet contains about 20 g/day dietary fibre (during the war it was 32–40 g/day). Metabolic studies show that fibre from cereals has a greater faecal bulking effect than that from fruit and vegetables. Increasing the fibre content of the diet is likely to reduce the absorption of minerals, e.g. calcium, iron and zinc but the magnitude of this effect depends on the mineral content of the diet, the nutritional state of the individual, the form in which fibre is ingested and the length of time on the diet (because adaptation occurs). For this reason it seems wise to suggest that extra dietary fibre should be derived from whole food which will ensure an increased intake of micro-nutrients.

The NACNE advised an increase in fibre consumption by the British population to a mean of 30 g a day over 15 years (i.e. by the turn of the century). Meanwhile before being able to give more specific recommendations nutritionists must await the results of detailed studies on the physiology, biochemistry and bacteriology of the colon in relation to food intake and other environmental factors in differing populations.

REFINED SUGAR

Relationship to obesity

Sugar has a particularly poor image with the proponents of 'healthy eating'. It is often described as empty calories, i.e. energy with no food value. On the other hand the food industry is well aware of its low cost, its purity, its keeping qualities and the palatability which it adds to processed foods.

Sugar was first cultivated over 2000 years ago in the Far East. It was not introduced into Britain in quantity until the 18th century, and its use only became widespread a century ago when the import duty was lifted.

The British like sweet food. National statistics show a consumption of 100 lb (45 kg) of refined sugar a year per head of population (80–85% as sucrose). Since the war there has been a substantial fall in the household purchase of packet sugar but this change has been counterbalanced by an increased consumption of convenience foods many of which contain sugar.

It is reasonable to believe that a sweet tooth predisposes to obesity although this would be hard to prove. Experiments on laboratory animals supports show that free access to a cafeteria diet leads to a greater intake of calories than the provision of unlimited supplies of animal chow. On the other hand, dietary studies have shown that slim active people often have a high sugar intake. Sometimes they appear to use sugar as a means of satisfying short-term energy needs. Thus a South African cane cutter moving 5–7 tons of cane a day may eat more than 300 g sugar a day. He is not obese, nor diabetic and he has a low serum cholesterol (about 150 mg/dl or 4.0 mmol/l).

Relationship to dental caries

Sugar is directly responsible for dental decay. It initiates the dissolution of enamel and allows the development of plaque built up by bacteria (especially *Streptococcus mutans*) from insoluble polymers of glucose and fructose (dextrans and levans). Monosaccharides can penetrate the plaque and are fermented to lactic acid which further erodes the enamel exposing the dentine and tooth pulp to attack.

Although sugar intake has changed little over the past 10–15 years there has been a big reduction in the prevalence of dental caries. The average number of decayed deciduous teeth in 5-year-olds living in England and Wales fell from 3.3 in 1973 to 1.6 in 1983; for permanent teeth in 15-year-olds the figures are 8.4 (1973) and 5.6 (1983) (Fig. 6.2). There are, however, big regional variations. The Scottish and

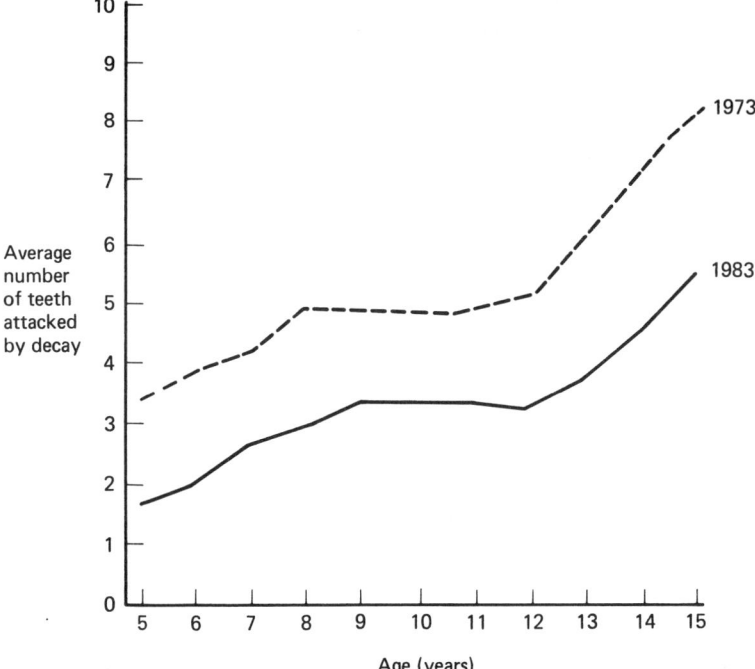

Figure 6.2 Average number of teeth with known decay for children of different ages in England and Wales (1973–1983).

Northern Irish figures are lagging a decade or more behind those of England, and the affluent south-east is faring better than the north and west of England. Changes reflect the use of fluoride-containing toothpaste and improved dental care (cleaning of teeth, use of fissure sealants by dentists) rather than a change in sugar consumption.

Attractive snack foods are often rich in fat and sugars. They provide concentrated energy but little in the way of other nutrients and are sometimes termed 'junk' foods. Breakfast cereals may contain more than 50% sugar (e.g. Sugar Puffs), cakes and biscuits more than 40%

and some soft drinks more than 25% (Ribena as much as 60%). There is little harm in consuming small quantities of such foods as snacks but if they are used to replace meals then the nutrient content of the diet as a whole is diluted.

In the production of dental caries the amount of refined carbohydrate consumed is much less important than its nature and the frequency of eating. Sticky foods adhering to teeth and staying in crevices provide an important substrate for bacteria. The need for more education in these simple facts is underlined by the parental response to questions in the recent OPCS survey (1983); 75% of parents blamed the eating of sweets for dental caries. Yet of the same respondents only 40% rated the avoidance of sweet foods as very important. Cleaning teeth regularly (75%) was regarded as the best means of prevention.

It is estimated that refined sugar consumption should fall to less than 35 lb (15–75 kg)/head/year as a public health measure to try to eliminate dental caries. Against this evidence the NACNE proposals appear to be conservative (see Table 1.8, p. 11). More work is needed, however, to determine the relative qualities of the many foods which contain sugar. A toffee containing 10 g of sugar may be very different from a similar amount in a helping of baked beans.

ALCOHOL

Over the past 20 years in Britain alcohol intake has increased 60–70%. Beer remains the most popular drink but the increase in intake per head of population (aged 15 years and over) has been relatively small (25%) compared with a 5–6-fold increase in wine drinking and a 2-fold increase in the taking of spirits (Fig. 6.3). Beer has increased in price relative to the all-price index but spirits have become considerably cheaper (Fig. 6.3b). The growth in alcohol consumption is reflected in the increasing prevalence of alcohol-related diseases. Groups at special risk include publicans, the unemployed, travelling business men and members of the medical profession. Women tolerate alcohol less well

Figure 6.3a, b and c National expenditure, price indices and consumption of alcohol in England and Wales (1960–1985). (Data taken from the *Annual Abstract of Statistics*. London: HMSO.)

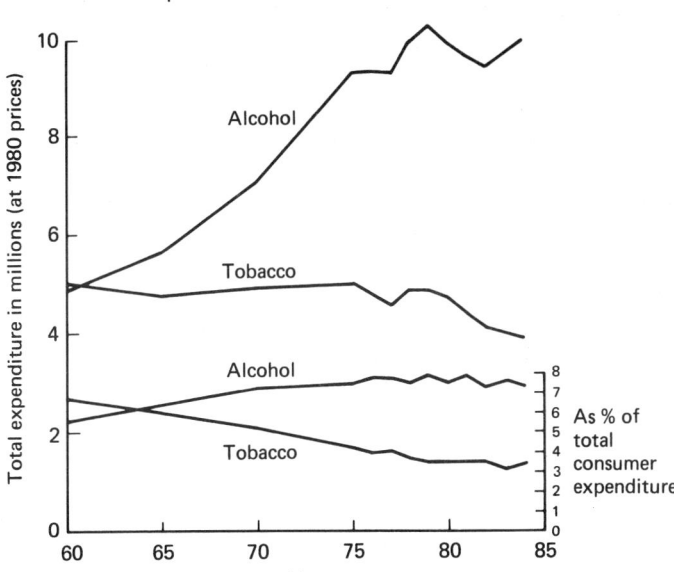

Figure 6.3a

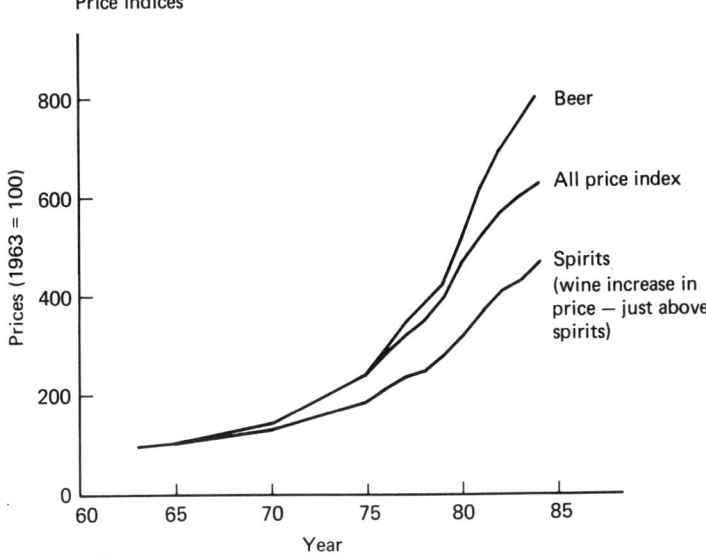

Figure 6.3b

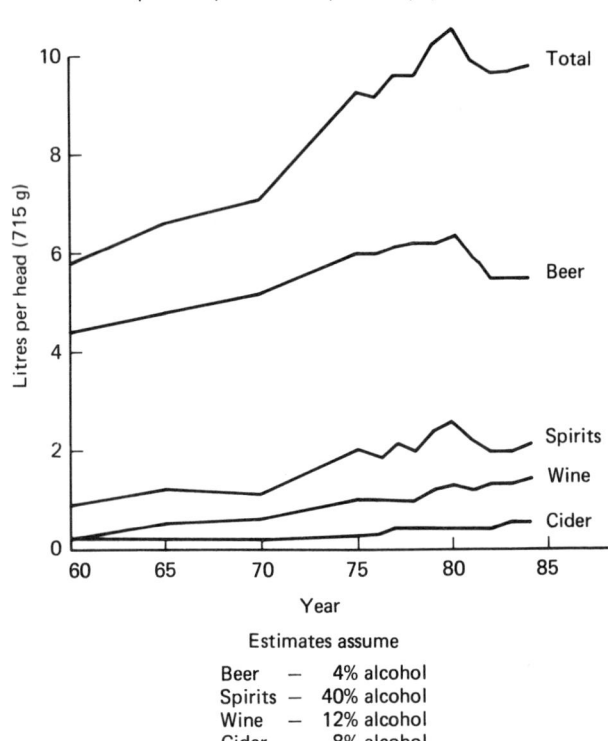

Figure 6.3c

than men and often present with advanced disease after a prolonged period of drinking excessively at home.

Records of HM Customs and Excise show that in the year 1700, alcohol intake in Britain (mainly as ale) was twice as great as it is today. Although we have no means of knowing the prevalence of alcohol-related disease contemporary descriptions suggest that gout and dropsy were common conditions.

Be that as it may, alcohol is an important risk factor in present-day society and should be recognized as such. Over recent years successive governments have been reluctant to attempt fiscal control. The cost of alcohol in relation to disposable income has fallen: for spirits by more than 50% and to a greater extent for wine than for beer (Fig. 6.3b). In 1960 more was spent on cigarettes than alcohol. By 1980 expenditure

Diet and the Epidemiology of Disease

on alcohol had doubled whereas that on tobacco had started to fall. (Fig. 6.3a). More recent figures suggest that the consumption of alcohol may have reached a plateau but the prevalence of alcohol-related disease appears to be increasing. The temperate may be drinking less and the intemperate more. Clearly there is an urgent need to help those at risk.

FURTHER READING

General

Doll R., scientific editor. (1984). The geography of disease. *Brit. Med. Bull*; **40**(4): 307–408.
Howe P. S., ed. (1981). *Basic Nutrition in Health and Disease*. Philadelphia: W. B. Saunders.
Katch F. I., McArdle W. D. (1983). *Nutrition, Weight Control and Exercise*. Philadelphia: Lea and Febiger.
McArdle W. D., Katch F. I., Katch V. L. (1981). *Exercise Physiology: energy, nutrition and physical performance*. Philadelphia: Lea and Febiger.
Walker R. P. (1983). 'Advance of today . . . the discarded or derided dogma of tomorrow?' *Amer. J. Clin. Nut*; **38**: 148–51.

Fat and cholesterol

Burch P. R. J. (1980). Ischaemic heart disease: epidemiology. Risk factors and causes. *Cardiovasc. Res*; **14**: 307–38.
Council on Foods and Nutrition. (1959). Symposium on significance of lowered cholesterol levels. *J. Amer. Med. Assoc*; **170**: 2198–203.
MRFIT Group. (1982). Multiple risk factor intervention trial: risk factor changes and mortality results. *JAMA*; **248**: 1465–77.
NIH Consensus Conference. (1984). *Lowering Blood Cholesterol to Prevent Heart Disease*. (Available from Office of Medical Applications of Research, National Institutes of Health, Building 1, Room 216, Bethesda, Maryland 20892, USA.)
Oliver M. F. (1985). Strategies for preventing coronary heart disease. *Nut. Rev*; **43**: 257–62.

Salt

Brown J. J., Lever A. F., Robertson J. I. S., Semple P. F. (1984). Should dietary sodium by reduced? The sceptics position. *Quart. J. Med*; **53**: 427–37.
Parrott-Garcia M., McCarron D. A. (1984). Calcium and hypertension. *Nut. Rev*; **42**: 205–43.
Symposium. (1979). Report of the Task Force relating six dietary factors to the nation's health. *Amer. J. Clin. Nut*; **32**: 2621–748.

Fibre

Burkitt D. P., Trowell H. C., eds. (1981). *Western Diseases: their emergence and prevention*. London: Edward Arnold.

Cleave T. L. (1974). *The Saccharine Disease: conditions caused by the taking of refined carbohydrate such as sugar and white flour*. Bristol: John Wright.

Cleave T. L., Campbell G. D., Painter N. S. (1969). *Diabetes, Coronary Thrombosis and the Saccharine Disease*. Bristol: John Wright.

Lane W. A. (1918). Some remarks on chronic intestinal stress. *Lancet*, 2: 416–17.

Royal College of Physicians. (1980). *Medical Aspects of Dietary Fibre: a report from the Royal College of Physicians*. London: Pitman Medical.

Spiller G. A., Kay R. M., eds. (1980). *Medical Aspects of Dietary Fiber*. New York: Plenum Press.

Trowell H., Burkitt D., Heaton K., eds. (1985). *Dietary Fibre, Fibre-depleted Foods and Disease*. London: Academic Press.

Walker A. R. P. (1971). Diet, bowel motility, faeces composition and colonic cancer. *S. Afr. Med. J*; 45: 377–9.

Walker A. R. P., Holdsworth C. M., Walker E. J. (1971). Investigation on the consumption of sugar by South African populations. *S. Afr. Med. J*; 45: 516–24.

Dental caries

Cohen B. (1979). Scientific basis for the prevention of caries and periodontal disease. *Proc. Roy. Soc. Med*; 74: 262–6.

Office of Population Censuses and Surveys (OPCS). (1983). *Children's Dental Health*. (OPCS monitor SS 83/2). London: OPCS.

Todd J. E., Dodd T. (1985). *Child Dental Health in the UK 1983*. London: HMSO.

Alcohol

Sherlock S., ed. (1982). Alcohol and disease. *Brit. Med. Bull*; 38(1): 1–114.

Chapter

7

The Future of Clinical Nutrition

CLINICAL NUTRITION IN HOSPITAL PRACTICE • GENERAL PRACTICE • COMMUNITY HEALTH • RESEARCH IN CLINICAL NUTRITION • FURTHER READING

Clinical nutrition cuts across all branches of medical practice. It has implications for all age-groups and for all body systems. It is a subject for the generalist rather than the specialist and for this reason it fails to make an impact as an independent clinical discipline.

In an analogous way, in the preclinical sciences, human nutrition also tends to be an orphan subject. The nutritionist needs a good working knowledge of the basic sciences, especially biochemistry and physiology, yet must also be reasonably well versed in psychology, sociology and epidemiology, and have some acquaintance with the principles of food science and technology.

CLINICAL NUTRITION IN HOSPITAL PRACTICE

In Britain clinical nutrition is not recognized as a specialist subject in schemes for higher medical training. In the US, where sub-specialization is more developed and multi-disciplinary care of patients is more common, hospital-based specialists in clinical nutrition are appointed and act on a consultative basis. They are usually concerned primarily with providing systems of nutritional support. In private practice the specialist in nutrition may deal solely with obese subjects and is called a bariatrician! Thus in the US clinical nutrition as a coherent discipline is limited in scope. This reflects a system with a high degree of specialization based on organ pathology.

In Sweden postgraduate training programmes in clinical nutrition are superimposed on specialty interests (internal medicine, endocrinology, gastroenterology, nephrology, long-term care, paediatrics, community medicine). The specialist in clinical nutrition does not have beds (except perhaps in a metabolic unit), but may have wide responsibilities within the hospital. These include:

Organizing a nutrition support service.
Providing a consultation service for nutritional assessment.
Controlling the dietetic service (including the interpretation of all requests).
Undertaking out-patient clinics to provide dietary advice for the management of patients with a variety of disorders.
Liaising with the department of clinical chemistry.

Elsewhere a different approach has been used to try to establish clinical nutrition in hospital practice. University based departments of human nutrition have been developed in some centres, e.g. in Southampton in the UK and in Sydney in Australia. These units have clinical links and may have academic status within the department of clinical medicine. Such departments tend to be more concerned with teaching and research than with clinical practice.

From this brief review it is obvious that in spite of considerable effort over the past decade or more, the practising specialist in clinical nutrition remains a rare species with a weak image. In the UK general practitioners refer their patients to organ-based specialists, such as cardiologists and gastroenterologists. It has proved difficult to obtain widespread recognition for 'agent' based clinical specialties, such as clinical pharmacology and clinical immunology.

In clinical nutrition the status of the specialist is eroded still further by the advertising pressure of commercal interests, by pressure groups who claim that diet is responsible for much degenerative and neoplastic disease and by publicists who use the popular media to great effect. Clinical scientists tend to shy away from nutritional problems. The questions posed are important but difficult to answer, and much of the published work is scientifically weak. A few years ago it seemed possible that the technical problems of providing artificial nutritional support would provide a disciplinary basis for clinical nutrition, as dialysis did for nephrology. Now this seems unlikely.

Thus the future remains uncertain. Specialist physicians are as effective as their clinical base allows. For clinical nutrition it seems that such a base can develop only out of one or more existing specialties. Perhaps a well established broadly-based specialty offers the most promising way forward. Paediatricians and geriatricians are tied to their age-related groups (although there is a higher incidence of nutritional problems at the extremes of age); clinical biochemists and specialists in metabolic medicine are constrained by their laboratory backgrounds and the organ-based specialist is too narrowly interested, e.g. the cardiologist interested in lipid metabolism or the hepatologist interested in alcoholism.

The specialist in clinical nutrition may have most influence if he is a busy general physician (or surgeon). Clinical colleagues are more likely to trust and seek advice from a fellow clinician, and clinical students probably remember more of what they see at the bedside than what is taught in the classroom. In Britain some general physicians and surgeons have been appointed to posts with an interest in gastroenterology and clinical nutrition. They have developed nutrition teams to standardize the care of patients requiring artificial nutritional support and many have shown a special interest in one or more of the nutritional disorders described in Chapter 3. Physicians with an interest in endocrinology and diabetes mellitus provide an alternative source of expertise. Some have a special interest in patients with anorexia nervosa, obesity or hyperlipidaemia. Thus in present day hospital practice there are pointers for the clinicians with an interest in nutrition and intermediary metabolism to complement the roles of specialist gastroenterologists and specialist endocrinologists. Such posts are most likely to develop in large teaching hospitals and for their successful development those appointed should have a strong base in general internal medicine. Clinical nutrition specialists who have no ward base will find it difficult to influence the management of patients and to teach clinical students effectively.

GENERAL PRACTICE

General practitioners need to be well versed in the principles of dietetics if they are to satisfy the demands of their patients. 'What shall I eat, doctor?' is a common question and often, I suspect, one that gets no more than a cursory reply. Few practices have the services of a dietitian, and community dietitians are thinly spread (1/50 000 population). For the most part primary care is supplied through the traditional one-to-one patient–doctor contact. At this level the general practitioner must seek to cope with the common disorders which require dietary advice – obesity, diabetes mellitus, dyspepsia, non-specific abdominal disorders and feeding problems in infancy and childhood. In addition he has the opportunity of screening for hyperlipidaemia early diabetes and early alcoholism. He may also organize sessions for subjects with mild to moderate obesity either directly or through the help of a community dietitian (see p. 101).

In day-to-day practice the very young and the very old take up much of the time of the general practitioner. Dietary advice is frequently sought and the general practitioner may need to liaise closely with other members of the primary care team to ensure that the patient receives a consistent message. Health visitors are especially well aware of the interest of the general public in the dietary management of disease (Table 7.1).

Table 7.1 *The importance of nutrition: Topics people most often wish to discuss with health visitors*

In relation to children <5 years		In relation to the elderly	
Diet	58	Home help	55
Physical development	50	Specific illness	50
Immunisation	44	Diet	39
Postnatal care	40	General health	38
Emotional problems	36	Adjusting to illness	35
General health	32	Nursing care	26
Housing	19	Housing	19
Other	130	Other	89

From: Clark J. (1973). *A Descriptive Analysis of Health Visiting in Berkshire.* London: Royal College of Nursing.

The challenge for the general practitioner is not only to detect and treat disease but to help individuals attain and maintain good health by their own efforts. The practitioner has to formulate his own attitudes to the role of nutrition in achieving these aims. And he must do this in the face of expert advice which is characterized by disagreements and inconsistencies. The future of general medicine appears to show an increasing trend towards teamwork. Dietitians may come to play a major part interpreting the advice of nutrition scientists, the exhortations of official bodies and the pressures of the food industry. The

The Future of Clinical Nutrition

general practitioner, however, will remain the focus for care and advice. In order to function well he will need to keep up with the information his patients receive from the media on nutrition and disease.

COMMUNITY HEALTH

During the first half of this century nutrition was an important part of public health because a significant proportion of the population was underfed. With the outbreak of war food was rationed but became available at a price all could afford. This led to a dramatic improvement in the health of the poor. Since the war, community nutrition has received relatively little attention in Britain. Now, however, there is a surge of interest. In 1973 the Secretary of State for Social Services (Sir Keith Joseph) set up a working party including representatives of the DHSS, the Health Education Council and the British Nutrition Foundation (funded by the food industry) with the task of satisfying 'the urgent need for . . . simple and accurate information on nutrition'. Progress was slow until 1979 when the working party recommended establishing a National Advisory Committee on Nutrition Education under the chairmanship of Professor J. N. Morris. The committee covered a wide range of interests with representatives of the DHSS; the Ministry of Agriculture, Fisheries and Food (MAFF); the British Nutrition Foundation; the Health Education Council and unaligned nutritional scientists. Advice must have been conflicting and it soon became apparent that progress would not be made without compromise. At this stage Professor W. P. James was asked to produce a document summarizing the 'broad scientific consensus'. This task was undertaken by a small group of nutritional scientists who used eight previously published reports (Table 7.2) as the basis for their document. They decided that their statement should be applicable to the whole population and that target figures had to be provided. By April 1981 the task was complete but many members of the committee wanted modifications. A time-scale for gradual change was suggested in order to take account of the possible adverse effects on agriculture and the food industry in the short term. The document was rewritten a fourth time.

By now 10 years had passed and the DHSS was still unable to satisfy 'the urgent need' identified by Sir Keith Joseph. On 3rd July 1983 the

Table 7.2 Reports used in preparing the Report of the National Advisory Committee for Nutrition Education (NACNE Report)

1. DHSS. (1979). Report on Health and Social Subjects, No. 15. *Recommended Daily Amounts of Food, Energy and Nutrients for Groups of People in the United Kingdom.* London: HMSO.
2. DHSS. (1978). *Prevention and Health—Eating for Health.* London: HMSO.
3. DHSS. (1974). Report on Health and Social Subjects No. 7. *Diet and Coronary Heart Disease.* London: HMSO.
4. RCP and British Cardiac Society. (1976). Prevention of coronary heart disease. *J. Roy. Coll. Phys.*; **10**: 213–75.
5. RCP. (1981). *Report on Medical Aspects of Dietary Fibre.* London: Royal College of Physicians.
6. DHSS. (1981). *Prevention and Health. Avoiding Heart Attacks.* London: HMSO.
7. RCP. (1983). Obesity. *J. Roy. Coll. Phys.*; **17**: 3–58.
8. DHSS. (1981). Report on Health and Social Subjects, No. 23. *Committee on Medical Aspects of Food Policy Nutritional Aspects of Bread and Flour.* London: HMSO.

NACNE Report. (1983). *Ad hoc* working party of National Advisory Committee for Nutrition Education. *Proposals for Nutritional Guidelines for Health Education in Britain.* London: Health Education Council.

Sunday Times ran a lead story suggesting that industrial interests had constrained the DHSS not to publish the NACNE document. Later that year it was released not by the DHSS but by the Health Education Council as 'a discussion paper on Proposals for Nutritional Guidelines for Health Education in Britain prepared by the National Advisory Committee on Nutrition Education by an *ad hoc* working party under the chairmanship of Professor W. P. James'.

The inevitable happened. The delays in producing official information together with the pressure of publicists gave the document a status which almost certainly was not intended by the majority of the National Advisory Committee. Within a few months a book was published entitled *The Food Scandal* (see Walker and Cannon, 1984) and the *Lancet* (see Editorial, 1983) was printing statements on 'implementing the NACNE report'. Discussion had given way to action, community health physicians were drawn into the mainstream and the media profited from the opportunity to publicize any aspect

The Future of Clinical Nutrition

which would excite public interest ('government cover-up', 'industrial pressure', 'controlling the modern epidemics', 'the new foods', 'cooking for health' and so on).

Clearly, however, the time was ripe for change. As long ago as 1943 an International Food Conference at Hot Springs, Virginia recommended the establishment of national food and nutritional policies. It was implied that such policies should involve more than the provision of 'wholesome' food and clean water. Epidemiological observations indicated associations between diet and chronic disease (see Chapter 5). These were not to be ignored.

In fact Norway was the only country to establish a national food and nutrition policy. The scale has been ambitious and the results sufficiently encouraging for the planners and politicians to continue to press for the achievement of the original goals (Table 7.3).

Today, in Britain, community health physicians must assess the evidence critically; they will be involved in advising on changes and in the assessment of the effects of such changes. This is an enormous brief. None of the chronic diseases – coronary artery disease, stroke, hypertension, diabetes and cancer – are the result of a single cause. Diet is almost certainly a contributory factor but its importance is uncertain. The lag period between interventional change and apparent effect may be prolonged (even up to 30 years). Modifying diet in adult life may be too late to affect outcome. Moreover compliance with dietary recommendations can be monitored only in a broad sense and only against a background of other factors which are also changing (e.g. smoking and exercise).

Scientists vary in their acceptance of epidemiological evidence. It is probable that experimental data will not become available to answer many of the questions posed. Thus it is necessary to decide whether epidemiological associations are aetiologically significant (Table 7.4). This has been done for smoking. Today few clinicians or scientists would deny a causative correlation with lung and heart pathology even though proof is not absolute. Many important issues of public policy have to be decided on incomplete evidence (see Table 7.5).

On balance professional opinion favours the view that a modification of Western diets along the lines of the NACNE document will reduce the incidence of the major chronic diseases in middle age. Americans have taken steps to modify their diet in these directions and the incidence of coronary heart disease has fallen. Although it is not possible to prove cause and effect the evidence is persuasive.

Table 7.3 *Features of Norwegian food policy* (McLaren, 1983)

Goals
1. Improve individual health
   Reduce intake of fat (to 35%)
   Increase intake of carbohydrate (cereals and potatoes)
   Reduce ratio of saturated fatty acids: polyunsaturated fatty acids (from >3:1 to 2:1)
2. Provide farm workers with secure and satisfactory living
3. To meet recommendations of FAO (greater self-sufficiency, help economically-weaker areas, make more effective use of national resources)

Note: Food to be presented as sources of nutrition rather than as commodities.

Means of implementing
1. Facilitating (enabling) means, e.g. subsidies
2. Regulating means: sanctions, quotas, price regulations
3. Education and information

Administration
Coordinating framework (Office of Nutrition in Ministry of Social Affairs)

Time scale
15 years—1975 to 1990

Trends—the first 5 years
Unexpected big rise in the fast food market ('chips and Coke')
Found difficult to control retail prices
Positive signs
   Decrease in consumption of edible fats
   Increase in consumption of cereals
   Decline in fish consumption halted
Negative signs
   Decreased potato consumption
   Increased sugar consumption

Changes
Results overall regarded as sufficiently encouraging to continue to try to achieve goals. More emphasis to be given to education and personal responsibility for health.

McLaren D. S., ed. (1983). *Nutrition in the Community: a critical look at nutrition policy, planning and programmes.* New York: John Wiley.

Satisfactory data on the effect of a prudent diet on other major chronic disorders (see Tables 6.1, 6.2 and 6.4) are not available.

Table 7.4 *Factors to consider in assessing epidemiological associations*

An epidemiological association is more likely to have aetiological significance if statistically:

1. it can be shown to be independent of other factors;
2. it is strong (high R value);
3. it shows a graded response;

and if it is consistent with other criteria such as:

1. Repeated studies giving similar results.
2. A reasonable temporal sequence for the proposed relationship.
3. Support from clinical observations and experimental findings.
4. The findings can be used successfully to make predictions.

Nevertheless, changes in diet similar to those described in the NACNE document (see Table 1.8) have been accepted by most Health Authorities in affluent countries despite some powerful opposition (Tables 7.5, 7.6). It seems unlikely that these changes could be seriously harmful

Table 7.5 *Examples of lines of evidence used to support the need for a national food policy*

Evidence used by protagonists	Reply by antagonists
Epidemiological correlations of diet and disease	Cause and effect not demonstrable
Prospective studies which reveal major risk factors	Relative importance of factors uncertain
Retrospective studies on effects of changes in life-style	Variables uncontrolled
Intervention studies	Give equivocal results (e.g. MRFIT). Reduction in morbidity from one cause counter-balanced by increase in other causes

although the somewhat cynical view that they will do no more than change the pattern of disease may prove to be correct. Time will tell. Meanwhile community physicians must do their best to monitor the effects of dietary change and to provide accurate data by which to judge the results.

Table 7.6 Examples of arguments used to oppose a national food policy

Argument	Reply
Proposed changes irrelevant to health of the majority. Require research to identify those at most risk	Total figures of morbidity/mortality arise mainly from the many at mild-moderate risk; not the few at high risk
Proposed levels of nutrient intake not supported by firm scientific data	Evidence is epidemiological—thus estimates have to be made on best available guidelines
More and better controlled trials needed—not half-baked decisions	Agree need for trials but decisions cannot be deferred indefinitely. Otherwise leave solely to the food industry
Healthy immortality is not achievable. Public need to know likely alternatives—?cancer, ?senile dementia, ?total frailty	The aim of a national nutrition policy is to reduce morbidity in the prime of life
Proposals mean sacrificing foods people like—an intolerable interference with freedom	Freedom is incomplete—tastes are acquired and in many cases nurtured by skilful advertising

RESEARCH IN CLINICAL NUTRITION

In nutrition most of the major steps forward have been made by chemists and biochemists. The geneology has been traced by Olsen (1978). Research in clinical nutrition entered its first phase at the beginning of the century when Voit in Germany and Atwater in the USA explored energy metabolism and body protein needs. The next phase was established by physician-scientists. Christian Eijkman of Utrecht showed that beri-beri was a deficiency disease and Frederick Hopkins from Cambridge enunciated the general concept that animals could not live by protein, fat, carbohydrate and minerals alone. They were jointly awarded the Nobel prize. Vitamins were there to be discovered. It was a period of intense excitement with clear scientific aims. Scientists had to identify the essential nutrients: their requirements for maintenance, growth and development, and their distribution in foods. With such knowledge it would be possible to define

The Future of Clinical Nutrition

nutritionally adequate diets. The task was completed by the end of the Second World War. The aims had been largely achieved but by then it was clear that it was not sufficient just to define dietary allowances. There were too many loose ends. Mankind is not a laboratory animal. Individuals are biologically very different from one another. Their needs differ, their abilities to adapt to differing levels of nutrient intake are ill-understood, and requirements for one nutrient may be markedly influenced by other dietary factors. Thus diet is more than a simple mixture of 50 or so nutrients (see Table 1.1). Much remains to be learned about their uptake and meabolism. The techniques of the cell biologist and enzymologist should help solve many of the outstanding issues.

After the Second World War many clinicians interested in nutrition concentrated on the problems of protein-calorie malnutrition. The nature of Kwashiorkor was defined and evidence has subsequently accumulated about the energy needs of mankind. New techniques of measuring energy output in the free-living state over prolonged periods are revolutionizing previous concepts. Mankind can live healthily on considerably fewer calories than the estimates of Voit and Atwater.

Today, however, the major research interest in clinical nutrition arises from the need for a better understanding of the epidemiology of chronic disease in wealthy industrialized countries. The concepts of 'medical disorders of affluent societies', 'the saccharine disease', and 'nutrition, lipids and coronary heart disease' require critical examination. Many of the findings of epidemiologists and even more of their conclusions have been hotly disputed by clinical scientists. In part this reflects attitudes dependent on the experimental approach of basic science rather than those based on observation and deduction (as are used in the study of subjects like astronomy and geology), and in part a medical training which concentrates on diagnosis and treatment rather than on preventive medicine and public health. There is clearly much to be done to try to solve the present contradictions and confusions concerning the aetiology of the chronic diseases which affect mankind in middle age. At the same time a tentative start has been made to try to identify the nutritional factors which may influence the ageing process.

Thus the opportunities for research in mainline nutritional science are considerable, but clinicians must be prepared to learn scientific skills in subjects outside clinical medicine if they are to be involved in major contributions.

And what of the future? Perhaps the most exciting developments will come from an examination of biological problems at a molecular level. The identification of deleterious genetic material and the study of food components and essential nutrients as factors in the control of gene expression may have a profound effect on clinical nutrition (Fig. 7.1).

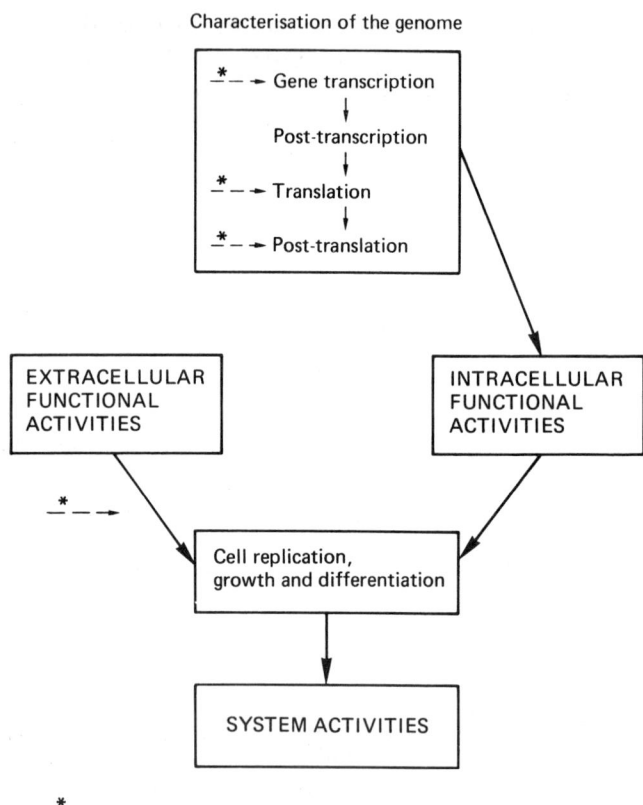

Figure 7.1 Molecular biology. From genome to organ function: The arrows show points at which nutritional factors may operate.

Vitamin A provides an example of the new science. The role of retinoids in lipid-linked carbohydrate transport and as components of visual purple are well known. In addition vitamin A status has been linked to the aetiology of cancer by somewhat uncertain epidemiological studies. Further understanding may come from the techniques of molecular biology. These have provided a completely new perspective on the effect of retinoids on the expression of proteins in epithelial cells. Retinoids are capable of activating and suppressing the transcription of genes and may act as nuclear mediators of cell differentiation. This is in contrast to the effects of most vitamins and essential minerals, which appear to act as enzyme cofactors in post-translational regulatory systems. The ability to execute metabolic reactions may be controlled by the enzymatic modification of amino acids in proteins. Thus vitamin A, ascorbic acid, copper, zinc and magnesium affect the formation of glycoproteins which in turn affect skeletal growth in experimental animals. Thus nutrition scientists have now to explore the molecular action and interaction of the essential nutrients defined two generations ago.

Meanwhile as the genetic code is unravelled it may become possible to identify individuals likely to develop atheroma, to become obese, or to suffer the effects of hypertension. This would make the present clumsy attempts to manipulate the diet of whole populations of much less significance. The starting point may be the eagerly awaited recognition of the gene for the production of low-density lipoprotein receptors and the identification of the defect in subjects with familial hypercholesterolaemia. This could be a major step forward in the realization of the dream of matching nutrition to genetic potential. Clinical nutritionists must be ready to meet the challenge.

FURTHER READING

Editorial. (1983). Are 'wholesome' food and water good enough? *Lancet*; 2: 715–16.
Hegsted D. M. (1985). Nutrition: the changing scene. *Nut. Rev*; 43: 357–67.
Masaro E. J. (1985). Nutrition and ageing – a current assessment. *J. Nut*; 115: 842–8.
McLaren D. S., ed. (1983). *Nutrition in the Community: a critical look at nutrition policy, planning and programmes*. New York: John Wiley.
Olson R. E. (1978). Clinical nutrition, and interface between human ecology and internal medicine. *Nut. Rev*; 36: 161–77.
Rucker R., Tinker D. (1986). Critical review: the role of nutrition in gene expression. *J. Nut*; 116: 177–89.
Walker C., Cannon G. (1984). *The Food Scandal: what's wrong with the British diet and how to put it right*. London: Century.

Appendix 1

General Further Reading

REFERENCE RESOURCE

Paul A. A., Southgate D. A. (1978). *McCance and Widdowson: The Composition of Food*. Amsterdam, London: Elsevier.

Woolfson A. M. J., ed. (1986). *Biochemistry of Hospital Nutrition*. Edinburgh: Churchill Livingstone.

TEXTBOOKS

Bender A. E., Bender D. A. (1982). *Nutrition for Medical Students*. New York, Chichester: John Wiley.
(Good review of nutritional principles which are then applied to the broader problems facing both developing countries and affluent peoples.)

Dickerson J. W. T., Lee H. A. (1978). *Nutrition in the Clinical Management of Disease*. London: Edward Arnold.
(A detailed study of clinical disorders by 17 authors – now somewhat dated; plentiful references.)

Feldman E. B., ed. (1983). *Nutrition in the Middle and Later Years*. Bristol: John Wright.
(An interesting American survey.)

Goodhart R. S., Shils M. E. (1980). *Modern Nutrition in Health and Disease*, 6th edn. Philadelphia: Lea and Febiger.
(Major American text on nutritional science.)

Kemm J. R., ed. (1985). *Vitamin Deficiency in the Elderly*. Oxford: Blackwell Scientific Publications.
(A good simple review.)

McLaren D. S., ed. (1982). *Textbook of Paediatric Nutrition*. Edinburgh: Churchill Livingstone.
(A useful specialist text.)

Passmore R., Eastwood M. A. (1986). *Human Nutrition and Dietetics*, 8th edn. Edinburgh: Churchill Livingstone.
(Classic British text on human nutrition recently updated.)

General Further Reading

Taylor K. B., Anthony L. E. (1983). *Clinical Nutrition*. New York: McGraw-Hill.
(A good introduction to the subject.)
Walker A., Hendricks K. (1985). *Manual of Paediatric Nutrition*. Philadelphia: W. B. Saunders Co.
(A concise practical reference manual.)
Walser M., Imbembo A. L., Margolis A., Elfert G. A. (1985). *Nutritional Management*. Philadelphia: W. B. Saunders Co.
(A useful book which attempts to bridge the gap between clinicians and dieticians.)
Weinsier R. L., Butterworth C. E., Jr. (1981). *Handbook of Clinical Nutrition*. St Louis, Missouri: C. V. Mosby Co.
(Excellent concise coverage of most clinical topics.)

SERIES

Advances in Nutrition Research (1977ff). New York: Plenum Press.
Contemporary Issues in Clinical Nutrition (1980ff). New York: Churchill Livingstone.
Annual Review of Nutrition (1981ff). California: Annual Reviews Inc.
NIH Consensus Conferences (available from Office of Medical Applications of Research, National Institutes of Health, Building 1, Room 216, Bethesda, Maryland, 20892, USA.)

JOURNALS

American Journal of Clinical Nutrition (Journal of the American Society for Clinical Nutrition)
Human Nutrition: Clinical Nutrition (British publication paired with Human Nutrition: Applied Nutrition)
Journal of Parenteral and Enteral Nutrition (Journal of the American Society for Parenteral and Enteral Nutrition)
Nutritional Reviews (published by the Nutrition Foundation).

Appendix 2

Training and Career Opportunities

In Britain there are no clearly defined training programmes for clinicians or scientists who wish to make a career in clinical nutrition. Nevertheless opportunities for developing an interest in the subject are slowly expanding. Clinicians should seek employment in an appropriate centre (see below). Those with a primary degree in nutrition have the opportunity to define an area of special interest in relation to human pathology, and directors of nutrition research units should seek to interest basic scientists in nutritional problems.

DEGREE COURSES IN NUTRITION

Basic degree courses in nutrition

University of London (Kings College)
University of Southampton
University of Surrey
University of Dublin (Trinity College)
Polytechnic of North London
Robert Gordon's Institute of Technology, Aberdeen

Higher degree courses in nutrition

London School of Hygiene and Tropical Medicine (MSc in human nutrition)
Kings College, London (MSc in nutrition)
University of Aberdeen (MPhil Course)

Postgraduate diploma courses at London School of Hygiene and Tropical Medicine, Leeds Polytechnic and Queens College Strathclyde.

UNIVERSITY/HOSPITAL DEPARTMENTS WITH AN INTEREST IN CLINICAL NUTRITION

London
  Central Middlesex Hospital (Dept of Gastroenterology and Nutrition)
  London Hospital (Dept of Gastroenterology)
  Royal Free Hospital (Dept of Medicine)
  St Bartholomew's Hospital (Dept of Clinical Nutrition)
  St George's Hospital (Dept of Medicine)
  St Thomas's Hospital (The Rayne Institute)
Aberdeen (Dept of Medicine and Rowett Research Institute)
Belfast (Dept of Medicine, Royal Victoria Hospital)
Bristol (Dept of Medicine, Royal Infirmary)
Cambridge (Dept of Gastroenterology and Clinical Nutrition, Addenbrooke's Hospital)
Dublin (Dept of Clinical Medicine, St James's Hospital)
Dundee (Dept of Medicine, Ninewells Hospital)
Edinburgh (Gastroenterology Unit, Western General Hospital)
Glasgow (Gastroenterology Unit, Royal Infirmary)
Leeds (Dept of Medicine, St James's Hospital)
Manchester (Dept of Surgery, Hope Hospital, Salford)
Newcastle (Dept of Surgery, Royal Victoria Infirmary)
Oxford (Dept of Surgery, Radcliffe Infirmary)
Southampton (Dept of Human Nutrition).

RESEARCH INSTITUTES

Aberdeen (Rowett Research Institute)
Cambridge (MRC Dunn Nutrition Unit).

Index

A *see* vitamins
acute phase proteins 61 (table)
Addison's disease 179
adolescent growth 34–6
Africa
  diet 4–9
  disease 134, 169 (table), 180, 183, 184
  growth of children 30 (table), 35
  malnutrition 84–7
agriculture 7–10, 14
albumin, serum 59–62
alcohol 11
  disease 58 (table), 93, 109, 115–16, 122, 186–9
  fetal development 26–7
  intake in Britain 187 (fig.)
  nutrient deficiencies 73 (table), 74–5, 91–2, 95–8
allergy 126–30, 170 (table)
amenorrhoea 22, 48, 88
  menstruation 89
America 4–6 (tables and fig.), 8–9 (tables), 169 (table)
  height studies 29–30
  see also United States
anaemia 59, 63
  nutritional 79 (table), 88–92
  in pregnancy 23, 24
anecephaly 25
anorexia nervosa 48, 61, 87–8
anthropometry 27–30, 43–8, 52 (fig.), 55–7, 151 (table)
antidiuretic hormone 77
aphthous ulcers 71
appetite 38, 120
  drugs which suppress 98, 107–8
artificial diet 1, 2 (table)
  see also enteral feeding
ascorbic acid (vitamin C) 79, 92, 156
Asia 4–5 (table), 8–9 (table), 30 (table), 35, 134, 169 (table)
  see also Japan

Asian diet 24, 98 (table)
asthma 39–40, 127 (table)
atheromatous disease 109
  see also cardiac disease
Australasia 33, 177, 192

B12 *see* cobalamin
basal metabolic rate 7 (table), 101
beri-beri 1, 96, 200
biliary obstruction 123
biotin 79 (table), 165 (table)
birthweight 20–2
blood 63–5, 76
  see also anaemia, iron
body composition 42–82
  active tissue mass 54–65
  blood 63–5
  build 44–8
  circulating proteins 59–63
  chloride 77
  fat 48–9
  fluid 74–7
  minerals 71–4
  muscle 54–7
  protein 49–54
  skin, mucous membranes 70–1
  structure and function 43–4
  supporting tissues 65–70
  trace elements 78–80
  viscera 57–9
  vitamins 78–9
Body Mass Index 101 (table)
bone 51–2, 65–70, 92–5
  histology 69 (figs.)
  radiology 66, 68 (figs.)
bone marrow 64, 96
brain, growth and development, 31–3, 96
Britain *see* United Kingdom
bulimia 87

cadmium in pregnancy 22
calcium 71–2

Index

absorption 114 (table), 117, 135 (table), 137–8
  in bones 65–70, 93–5
  in diet 14, 95 (table), 98
  neural tube defect 25
  renal disease 125
calories *see* energy
cancer 38–9 (table), 58 (table), 89, 94
  and diet 168–9, 169 (table), 183
Candida infection 71
carbohydrate 133–5
  intravenous 153, 156, 157
cardiac disease 38–9 (tables)
  diet 170–9
  nutritional disorders 96, 100, 106, 109
  trends 173 (fig.)
caries *see* dental caries
central venous lines 162–3
children, growth in 26–40
  population differences 30 (table)
chloride 77, 117, 139–40
cholecalciferol (vitamin D) 67
  mineral absorption 72, 138
  myopathy 58 (table)
  osteomalacia 67–70, 94–5
  pregnancy 24
cholesterol 14, 18, 136
  anorexia nervosa 88
  diabetes 114
  fibre 121
  heart disease 109, 175–8
  hypercholesterolaemia 109–12, 203
  obesity 103
cholestyramine 112 (table), 116
chromium 80 (table)
cirrhosis of liver 123
clinical practice 15–18
clofibrate 112 (table)
cobalamin (vitamin B12) 64, 91–2, 97, 114 (table), 117–18, 150 (table), 156 (table)
codeine phosphate 148
coeliac disease 18 (table), 71, 73, 114 (table), 117, 119 (table)
  allergy 127 (table), 128
  anaemia 89–91
  diets for 119 (table)
  growth inhibition 38–9 (tables)
colitis 75 (table)
community health 194–200
connective tissue 70–1
constipation 122, 181
copper 80 (table), 92, 139, 156, 165 (table)
corneal arcus 109
coronary heart disease *see* cardiac disease, cholesterol
corticosteroids 40, 58 (table), 99 (table)
  calcium in bones 65

cow's milk protein intolerance 127
creatinine 55 (table), 56
Crohn's disease 39 (table), 71, 73, 114 (table), 120
  diet for 119 (table)
Cushing's syndrome 58 (table), 105
cystic fibrosis 18 (table), 38 (table), 120

dairy food consumption 13–14
dehydration 61 (table), 63, 74–6
dental caries 115, 170 (table), 184–6
dermatitis herpetiformis 128
development *see* growth
diabetes mellitus 38 (table), 75 (table), 105, 122, 123
  diet for 112–14
  hyperlipidaemia 109–11
dialysis 126
diarrhoea, severe 119–20
diet
  assessment 14–17
  deficiencies 97 (table)
  disease 170 (table)
  goals 9–14
  history 15–17
  intake 1–19
  low calorie liquid 97 (table), 107
  patterns in history 10–14
  proposals for change 11
diethylpropion 108
dietitian 17
digestion 133–40
disaccharidase deficiency 199 (table), 134–5
diuretics 74–5, 77, 99 (table)
diverticular disease 182
drugs
  effect on appetite 98, 108
  effect on growth 40, 47
  effect on nutrients 74–5, 89, 92, 98–99, 99 (table)
  treatment 107–8, 112, 115–16, 144, 148
  see also corticosteroids, hormones
dumping 116
dysphagia 115, 133

E *see* vitamins, tocopherol
elderly, food intake 134 (table)
electrolyte
  absorption 139–40
  body losses 159 (table)
  total parenteral nutrition 149–67, 152 (table), 158–9
encephalocoele 25
encephalopathy (hepatic) 123–4
endocrine disorders 75 (table), 101
energy
  efficiency of food 8 (table)

requirement 3, 7 (table), 154–7
sources 4–6 (tables and fig.), 153, 156–7
enteral feeding 134, 136, 140–9
   nutritional requirements 152
   tube feeding 143–9
enzyme systems 62, 75, 98
epidemiology of disease 168–89
   alcohol 186–9
   assessment 199 (table)
   cancer 168–9
   cardiac disease 170–9
   cholesterol and fat 175–8
   fibre and carbohydrate 180–3
   salt 178–9
   sugar 184–6
epilepsy 94
essential fatty acids 82, 114 (table), 151, 157, 164 (table)
Europe 4 (table), 6 (fig.), 8 (table), 169 (table), 177
   growth rate 30 (table), 35
   lactase deficiency 134
   neural tube defects 25–6
   see also United Kingdom
extracellular fluid 74–7

failure to thrive 38 (table), 39 (table)
fat
   body 48–51
      assessment 44 (table)
      pregnancy and lactation 20–1
   consumption 5 (table)
      absorption 135 (table), 136
      disease 122–3, 175–8
      NACNE advice 11 (table)
      total parenteral nutrition 156
   see also obesity
fatty liver 85–6, 97, 164 (table)
fenfluramine 107, 108
fetus
   fetal alcohol syndrome 26–7
   fetal growth 20–6
fibre 11 (table)
   disadvantages 122
   intestinal disease 120–2,
   related disorders 174 (table), 180–4
fluid 74–7
   dehydration 61 (table), 63, 74–6
   overhydration 76–7, 164
fluoride 93, 115, 156 (table), 175
folic acid 90–1
   assessment 64
   deficiency 62–4, 70–1, 91, 137, 165 (table)
      alcoholic 96–7
      brain growth 31
      intestine 114 (table), 117
      pregnancy 23–5

   renal disease 126
food
   allergy 126–30, 170 (table)
   calcium content 95
   categories 1
   consumption in the UK 12, 13 (table)
   energy efficiency 8 (table)
   faddism 97 (table)
   intolerance 16–18, 126–30
   junk 97 (table)
   labelling 11 (table)
   national policy 194–200
   world wide availability 3–10
Framingham Study 176
fructose intolerance 18 (table)

galactosaemia 18 (table)
gallstones 122–3, 170
gastric surgery 86–7, 114 (table), 116–17
gastroenteritis treatment 121
gastroenterostomy 133
gastrointestinal disorders 114–22
   diet 169–70 (tables), 180–4
   growth rate 38 (table), 40, 47
   malabsorption 73 (table), 75 (table), 117–20
   mineral deficiency 73, 75 (table), 89, 90
   nutritional support 140–67
   protein-energy malnutrition 86–7
   vitamin deficiency 67, 92, 114 (table)
   see also coeliac disease, constipation, Crohn's disease, diverticular disease, gastric surgery, irritable bowel, oesophageal disease, pancreatic disease, protein-losing enteropathy, resection of small intestine
general practitioners 193–5
genetic factors 18–19, 202–3
   body fat 48, 100
   disorders 18 (table)
   height 33–5
   hyperlipidaemia 109–11
   hypertension 178–9
   neural tube defect 25
geographical variation in diet 3–10, 25
Germany, growth study 35
glossitis 71, 91, 115
glucose 2 (table), 72
   tolerance 88, 123, 149
gluten sensitivity 127
glycaemia 112–13, 116, 149
glycine 85
goitre 1, 80 (table)
gout 109
government food policy 9–11, 194–200
growth 20–40
   adolescent 33, 34

Index

brain 31
charts 28, 29, 32, 37 (figs.)
child 26–40
fetal 20–6
impairment 36–40 (tables)
infant 30–3
optimal 33–5

haematology 63–5
haematinics 64
haemoglobin 63
hair 70 (table)
Harpenden longitudinal studies 29
health 195–200
height
  assessment 27–30, 44–7
  body composition 49–50 (tables)
  growth rate 30–2, 36–7
heparin 65
hepatic encephalopathy 123–4
hepatic secretory proteins 59–62
hepatitis 122
histamine 127
history 10–14, 22, 116, 171–2
  research 200–1
home parenteral nutrition 150–1, 159
homocystinuria 18 (table)
hormones
  anorexia nervosa 88
  and body fat 48
  circulating proteins 61 (table)
  growth 38, 40
  osteomalacia 67
  osteoporosis 94
  overhydration 77
hospital practice 42–3, 191–2
H2-receptor antagonists 115
hydroxycobalamin see cobalamin
hyperlipidaemia 96, 108–12, 114
  see cholesterol, hypertriglyceridaemia
hyperparathyroidism 67, 75 (table), 125
hypertension 178–9
hypertriglyceridaemia 122
hypoparathyroidism 72
hypothrombinaemia 123

Imodium 148
immune response 62, 127
infant growth 30–3
infection 38–9 (tables), 61, 63
intestine 117–22, 133
  see also gastrointestinal disorders
intravenous feeding 153–67
intrinsic factor 91
iodine 59 (table), 80 (table), 156 (table)
iron 88–90, 137–9
  assessment 61 (table), 63–4
    anaemia 88–90

body stores 89
brain growth 31
deficiency 1, 88–90
gastrointestinal 59 (table), 114 (table), 117, 135 (table)
pregnancy, 23, 25
skin 70–1
TPN 156
irritable bowel syndrome 119 (table), 127, 181–2
isoleucine 98

Japan 6 (fig.), 33, 35
  disease 169, 176–7, 183
jaundice 136

K see vitamins
kidney see renal disease
koilonychia 70 (table)
kwashiorkor 70 (table), 75 (table), 83–7, fig. 4.1, 4.2
kyphosis of the spine 45

labelling of food 11 (table)
laboratory monitoring 79 (table), 149, 150 (table)
lactase 18 (table), 127, 134
  milk intolerance 38 (table)
large intestine 120–2
lead in pregnancy 22
Leiner's disease 79 (table)
Leningrad, birth weight study 22
leukonychia 70 (table)
leukopenia 64
lipids 136, 156–7
  see also hyperlipidaemia
liver disease 61 (table), 77, 96, 122–4
Looser's zones 67–8
lysine 85, 98

macrobiotic diet 97 (table)
magnesium 71–5, 138
  in alcoholics 96
  gastrointestinal disease 114 (table), 135 (table)
  hypomagnesaemia 75 (table), 96, 164 (table)
  osteomalacia 67
  pregnancy 22
  treatment 75 (table)
malabsorption see gastrointestinal disorders
malnutrition see undernutrition
manganese 156 (table)
maple syrup urine disease 18 (table)
marasmus 83, 84, 86
margarine consumption 13 (fig.)
MCT (medium chain triglycerides) 136
meat consumption 13 (fig.)

menopause, osteoporosis in 94
menstruation 89
  amenorrhoea 22, 48, 88
metabolism, tests of 62 (table), 79 (table)
methionine 98
metoclopramide 115, 144
Metropolitan Life Insurance Company, bodyweight 46, 100
milk alkali syndrome 116
milk intolerance 38 (table), 127, 134
  lactase deficiency 18 (table)
minerals 71–5
  absorption 117, 137
  in alcoholics 97 (table)
  chemically defined diet 2 (table)
  NACNE advice 11 (table)
  special diets 97
  see also calcium, copper, fluoride, iron, magnesium, trace elements
molecular biology 202 (fig.)
molybdenum 80 (table)
MRFIT Study 169, 171 (table)
mucous membrane 70–1
muscle, skeletal 44 (table), 51 (table), 54–9
  biopsy 56
  function 56, 58 (table)
  mass 55 (table)
myopathy 56, 58–9, 95

nail changes 70 (table)
National Advisory Committee on Nutrition Education (NACNE) 9–11, 195–7
neural tube defects 25–6
neurological disorders 38 (table), 59 (table), 91
New York, growth study 21
niacin, nicotinic acid 79, 85, 112 (table), 156, 197
night blindness 79 (table)
nitrogen 53–4, 143, 155–8, 164
  balance 54, 143
Norwegian food policy 197–8
nutrition
  assessment 42–81
  disorders 83–131
  support 132–67
  team 166–7

obesity
  assessment of 106 (table)
  causes of 99–101
  complications 105 (table)
  in disease 18 (table), 109, 122
  drugs 108
  jaw wiring 107
  management 100–8
  metabolic assessment 105 (table)
  mortality 102
  prevalence 99
  refined sugar 184
  surgery for 107
  see also fat, body
oesophageal disease 115
oestrogen 94
omeprazole 115
oral replacement fluid 121
osteomalacia 67–70, 94–5, 123, 126 (table)
osteoporosis 65–7, 93–4
overhydration 76–7

Paget's disease 68, 94
pancreatic disease 38 (table), 96, 110–11 (tables), 120, 135, 136
pantothenate 2 (table), 152 (table), 156 (table)
Papua New Guinea, energy study 3
paracetamol poisoning 98
pellagra 79 (table), 85
phenylketonuria 18 (table), 127
phosphorus 72–3, 139
  in disease 59 (table), 67, 73 (table), 96, 125, 149, 164 (table)
  treatment 73 (table)
phytate 67, 138
potassium 52–3, 139–40
  in disease 59 (table), 88, 125
pre-albumin 61 (table)
pregnancy 20–6
  alcohol damage 26
  anaemia 89, 91
  circulating proteins 61 (table)
  neural tube defects 25–6
  specific nutrient deficiencies 23–4
  undernutrition 22
Pregnavite Forte F 25
preventive medicine 9–10, 194–200
protein
  absorption 135–6
  assessment of 49–54
  brain growth 31
  circulatory proteins 59–63
  deficiency 59 (table), 62 (table), 70 (table)
  hepatic secretory 59–62
  hypoproteinaemia 71, 117
  -losing enteropathy 119 (table)
  malnutrition 83–7
  renal disease 125
  sources 4–6 (tables and fig.)
protein-energy malnutrition (PEM) 83–7, 117, 120
  Kwashiorkor 84–7
  marasmus 83–4
  undernutrition 7–8
  visceral disorders 59 (table)
puberty 34–6

Index

pyridoxine *see* vitamin B6

Quetelet's Index 50 (fig.), 100–3

recommended dietary allowances (RDAs) 6, 11
renal disease 124–6
    circulating proteins 61 (table)
    growth inhibition 38–9 (tables)
    hypomagnesaemia 75 (table)
    hypophosphataemia 73 (table)
    rickets 94
    stones 170
research 200–3
resection of small intestine 114, 119 (table)
retinol *see* vitamin A
retinol-binding protein 61 (table)
riboflavin (vitamin B complex) 79, 156
rickets 67–70, 94–5
Ryle's tube 143–5, 149

salt
    absorption 117, 139–40
    in body fluids 74, 76–7
    liver disease 123
    hypertension 178–9
    NACNE advice 11 (table)
Scandinavia 26, 33, 192
scurvy 1, 70 (table), 79 (table), 81 (table), 92
seborrhoea 70 (table), 79 (table)
selenium 59 (table), 80 (table), 165 (table)
serum albumin 59–62
skeleton 51–2, 64–70, 92–5
skin 70–1
skinfold thickness assessment 27–30, 48–9, 52 (fig.), 57 (fig.)
skin-prick tests 62
small intestine 117–20, 133, 135 (table)
    diets for disorders of small intestine 119 (table)
    see also gastrointestinal disorders
smoking 93, 102–3, 171, 175
sodium 14, 77, 88, 125
    absorption 117, 139–40
spina bifida 25
stagnant loop syndrome 87, 120
stature 30, 33–40
    short stature 36 (table)
steatorrhoea 120
stomach 114–16
stomatitis 70 (table), 115
Stone Age diet 10–11
sucrose, NACNE advice 11 (table)
sugar, refined 180, 184–6

teeth 115, 170 (table), 184–6

thiamin (vitamin B complex) 79, 96, 97 (table), 156 (table)
thrombocytopenia 64
thyroid hormone 108
thyrotoxicosis 58 (table)
total parenteral nutrition (TPN) 149–67
    care of lines 162 (table)
    complications 160–5
    delivery systems 159–60
    at home 165–6
    intravenous 153–9
    metabolic problems 164 (table)
toxic food 126
trace elements 14, 92
    assessment 44 (table), 78–82
    deficiencies 22–5, 97 (table)
    total parenteral nutrition 156, 165 (table)
transferrin 61 (table), 64
triglycerides 109 (table), 136
tropical sprue 114 (table), 120
tryptophan 85, 98
tube feeding 143–9
tyrosinaemia 18 (table)

ulcers, mouth 71
undernutrition 6–8
    alcoholics 95–6
    assessment 78–82
    body function 58–9, 62
    elderly 134 (table)
    feeding 140–67
    growth 36–8
    hospital 132
    pregnancy 22–6, 31
    protein-energy 83–7
    on specific diets 96–8
United Kingdom
    alcohol 26, 186–9
    diet 12, 13 (figs.)
    energy requirements 3
    growth rate 28–9, 37
    health care 191–200
    heart disease 172–3, 177
    household consumption of food 12, 13 (figs.)
    intestinal disease 180–3
    lactase deficiency 134
    NACNE goals 11 (table)
    nutrient deficiency 1, 174–5
    sugar, refined 184–6
    wartime diet 71
United Nations World Conference on the Food Situation 3
United States
    cancer 169 (table)
    dietary goals (1977) 9
    growth of children 21, 33, 46
    heart disease 172, 176–7

hospital practice 191
intestinal disease 180, 183
urticaria 127

vanadium 80 (table)
vascular disease 170 (table)
vegan diet 92, 98
vegetable consumption 12 (fig.), 14
vegetarian diet 97–8
very low calorie diets 97 (table)
visceral function 44 (table), 57–9
vitamins
   A, vitamin 1, 59, 61 (table), 79 (table), 97 (table), 202–3
   absorption 117, 120, 133, 135
   alcoholics 96, 97 (table)
   ascorbic acid (vitamin C) 79, 92, 156
   assessment 44 (table), 78–9, 81
   B complex 59, 79, 85, 96–8, 112 (table), 156 (table), 197
   B12 see cobalamin
   blood 63–4
   C see ascorbic acid above
   chemical diet 2 (table)
   cholecalciferol (vitamin D)
     deficiency 92–4, 97 (table)
     mineral absorption 72, 138
     myopathy 58 (table)
     osteomalacia and rickets 67–70, 94–5
   circulating proteins 61 (table)
   cobalamin (vitamin B12) 64, 91–2, 97, 114 (table), 117–18, 150 (table), 156 (table)
   D see cholecalciferol above
   deficiency in diet 14, 62, 79 (table), 97 (table)
   E see tocopherol
   fat-soluble 24, 120, 123, 135–6
     see also A, D, E and K
   gastrointestinal disease 114 (table)
   integument 70–1
   K, vitamin 79, 123, 135, 156
   NACNE advice 11 (table)
   neural tube defect 25
   pregnancy 22–5
   pyridoxine (vitamin B6) 64, 92, 156 (table)
   renal disease 125–6
   research 202–3
   tocopherol, vitamin E 79
   total parenteral nutrition 156, 159, 165 (table)
   visceral disorders 59 (table)
   water-soluble 24, 137
     see also B complex, ascorbic acid (C)

war, second world 22, 116, 171–2
water
   absorption 117, 120, 139–40
   chemical diet 2 (table)
   dehydration 61 (table), 63, 74–6
   liver disease 123
   overhydration 76–7
   total parenteral nutrition 158–9
weight
   assessment 27–30, 44 (table), 46–8
   birth 20–1, 26
   body composition 49–51 (tables)
   growth 37 (table)
Wernicke–Korsakoff syndrome 79 (table), 96
wheat consumption 12 (fig.), 14
Williams, Cicely 84–5

xanthomata 109
xerophthalmia 1, 59 (table), 79 (table)

Zen macrobiotic diet 97 (table)
zinc
   absorption 139
   brain growth 31
   circulating protein 61 (table)
   deficiency 70 (table), 80 (table), 97 (table), 165 (table)
   gastrointestinal 114 (table)
   pregnancy 22, 23–4
   skin 70 (table)
   TPN 156 (table)
   visceral disorders 59 (table)